HOW TO

SOLVE

GENETICS

PROBLEMS

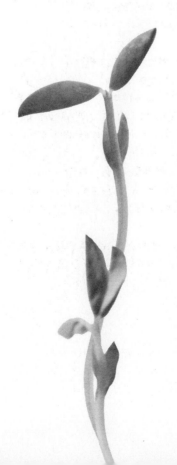

HOW TO
SOLVE
GENETICS
PROBLEMS

HARRY NICKLA, PH.D.
CREIGHTON UNIVERSITY

Benjamin Cummings

San Francisco Boston New York
Cape Town Hong Kong London Madrid Mexico City
Montreal Munich Paris Singapore Sydney Tokyo Toronto

Editor-in-Chief: Beth Wilbur
Executive Editor: Gary Carlson
Executive Director of Development: Deborah Gale
Editorial Assistant: Lindsay White
Managing Editor: Michael Early
Production Supervisor: Camille Herrera
Copyeditor: Joanna Dinsmore
Compositor and Illustrator: Harry Nickla
Cover Designer: Derek Bacchus
Manufacturing Buyer: Michael Penne
Executive Marketing Manager: Lauren Harp
Text and Cover printer: Edwards Brothers

Cover Photo Credits:
(DNA molecule) ©Mehau Kulyk / Science Photo Library;
(Pea sprout) ©Elena Elisseeva / Shutterstock.com

1 2 3 4 5 6 7 8 9 10—EB—10 09 08 07 06

Library of Congress Cataloging-in-Publication Data

Nickla, Harry, 1945-
  How to solve genetics problems / Harry Nickla.
    p. cm.
  Includes index.
  ISBN 978-0-321-55693-6 (pbk.)
  1. Genetics--Problems, exercises, etc. I. Title.
  QH440.3.N53 2010
  572.8076--dc22
                                          2009006792

Benjamin Cummings
  is an imprint of

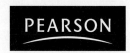

www.pearsonhighered.com

ISBN-13: 978-0-321-55693-6
ISBN-10: 0-321-55693-3

Contents

Preface

First:

Understanding genetics and solving genetics problems is achievable and within your grasp!

Second:

This ***is not*** another genetics text; there are many good ones available already.

This ***is not*** an outline series for genetics students. There are several good outline/problems books available already.

This ***is not*** a typical genetics workbook. Most texts include solved problems and websites with graded practice problems.

This book ***is*** written to complement your textbook and the lectures you will receive.

> ***The main purpose of this book is to tutor you in the development of problem-solving skills and, as a result, help you do well in genetics.***

This book was developed over decades of genetics instruction, individual tutoring, and countless review sessions with students at both introductory and advanced genetics levels.

The secondary purpose of this book is to help you develop skills necessary for success not only in genetics, but also in other courses and perhaps even life circumstances that require analytical thinking. It is designed to help you see trends, concepts, and patterns and apply each to the solution of problems or questions. Ultimately, this book should help you develop ways of thinking analytically.

There are a multitude of genetics texts and they all have common themes and expectations, whether they be in the content, the solved problem sections, or the chapter-ending questions and problems. This book presents ways of mastering content in an analytical framework, without repeating, those common themes.

> *...it's not the presentation, it's the mastery.*

Most genetics textbooks cover transmission, molecular, cytogenetic, and population genetics, in similar ways. The issue for the student is not so much the presentation of these topics, it's their mastery. While great lengths are taken to develop texts, study guides, CDs, workbooks, websites, and even professors, little is done to actually break down the processes by which one learns the subject.

This book will help you succeed by serving as a bridge between you and the subject matter. It will not help you memorize the subject. Rather, mastery and application of genetics concepts come through conceptual understanding and the ability to apply concepts when solving problems.

Many times, neither the teaching assistant nor the instructor has the time, patience, or capacity to be certain that every avenue is explored before a final low grade is assigned. That has been my motivation to write this book. It has been frustrating knowing that this kind of study aid was lacking for hundreds of students who could have been helped but never were.

A healthy disparity should exist between the subject matter covered in a course and the incoming knowledge of the student. Through struggle, conflict, and confusion, students are challenged to understand not only new subject matter, but also new ways of resolving problems. With incremental successes, students gain confidence and competence. Like many other courses of substance, genetics requires concentration, commitment, and perseverance. And while negotiating all three can be agonizing and demoralizing at times, each is worth achieving, not just because each represents a characteristic of an educated person, but also for the advantages they create in life.

This book can be your personal tutor to master basic classroom-level genetics.

> *Consider this book as your hired hand or personal tutor.*

Introduction

Does this sound familiar?

"I understood all the material but still failed your test."

"Nothing that I studied was on the test."

"This is the lowest grade I have ever received."

"I did fine on the practice tests you gave us, but I still failed your test."

"I studied all weekend and even pulled an all-nighter and still failed your test."

"I worked so hard, did all you said to do, spent weeks reading the chapters, doing the problems, working with old tests, memorizing your lectures and I still did poorly. What else can I do? Is there any extra credit?"

> *For each course you are taking, develop a realistic plan of study for each day, week, and semester. Stick with your plan!*
>
> *Study when there are no tests!*
>
> *Attend class; listen and think!*

The structure of this book is simple:

Each section (see below) should be addressed in the order that matches your class syllabus. While the order of subjects listed here may not reflect your particular course, the alignment should be obvious.

> Master each session as you encounter it in your course.

At the start of each section is a brief table of contents indicating the **concepts and processes** contained in that section, the **relative difficulty level of each question,** and the questions that relate to each concept/process. Be certain to finish all sections relating to a particular examination a couple of days before that examination. This will give you time to reconnect with the content of the course as provided by your instructor and/or textbook. It is very important that you not view this book as a review for a given test. This book will help you develop specific analytical skills, which should help you progress toward doing well on a variety of examinations.

Each question addresses at least one major concept or process. Each question addresses that core concept/process at different levels of difficulty, each requiring deeper understanding. Typically, genetics students will encounter more Level 1 and 2 questions on examinations; however, depending on the rigor of your course and the instructor, it is likely that sooner or later you will be expected to master Level 3 and 4 questions as well. Below is a description of question levels.

> Finish all relevant sessions several days before your exam.

Level 1: fairly straightforward, few complexities

Level 2: somewhat more involved than Level 1, perhaps with a slight twist

Level 3: more complex than Levels 1 and 2, but relatively straightforward, with a twist here and there

Level 4: considerable analysis required along with concept integration and manipulation

> See the patterns and develop an understanding.

There are no course or chapter outlines in this book. Its intent is to help you understand the most critical aspect of genetics --- approaches to problem solving. This book does not contain a comprehensive selection of solved problems. Rather, it contains a number of standard, often-used problems for each concept area that are analyzed sentence by sentence to help you develop understanding.

General organization of this book and each question: Throughout this book there are terms in **bold print**. Be certain that you achieve a complete understanding of these terms, as well as those given by your instructor or your textbook.

For each session, work all the questions at Levels 1 and 2. If you are enrolled in a course that focuses on the development of analytical, problem-solving, and critical thinking skills, you should also work questions at Levels 3 and 4.

Before the analysis of each question is a statement of the primary concepts and processes that each question encompasses.

Example:

> **Concepts/Processes in Question 1:** There are three primary aspects to this problem. First, there is one gene pair involved thereby, specifying a **monohybrid cross.** Second, the allele for normal pigmentation is **completely dominant** to the allele giving albinism. Third, each union of gametes is independent of previous unions and the **probability** of such unions can be determined. It is also important at this time to develop the use of **conventional genetic symbolism.**

The next section contains a complete analysis of each question, with sentence-by-sentence interpretations.

Analysis of each question

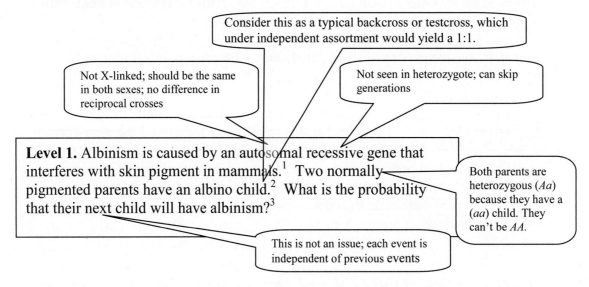

Sentence 1: Since a single trait is referred to, it is likely that a **monohybrid** cross is described....

Sentence 2: (complete and detailed explanation)

Sentence 3 and answer: (complete and detailed explanation)

This book examines major concepts and processes in a typical genetics course.

Session I: Chromosome Mechanics: *The physical basis of inheritance that establishes the mechanisms for transmission genetics*

Session II: Mendelian Genetics: *The processes by which traits are passed from parent to offspring*

Session III: Applications and Extensions of Mendelian Genetics: *A variety of conditions that influence the expression of genes*

Session IV: Linkage, Crossovers, and Mapping: *Consequences that arise when two or more genes are located on the same homologous chromosome pair*

Session V: Molecular Biology: DNA: *The chemical basis of inheritance*

Session VI: Molecular Biology: Techniques: *Methods of nucleic acid analysis*

Session VII: Molecular Biology: Pathways, Proteins, Transcription, Translation, and Mutation: *The expression and alteration of the genetic material*

Session VIII: Genetic Regulation in Prokaryotes: *The control of gene expression*

Session IX: Population Genetics: *The assessment of gene frequencies in populations*

Give yourself a chance at success:

Read all assigned materials before class
Attend each class
Do all the assigned problems
Attend review sessions if available
Study when there are no tests
Establish a realistic study schedule and stick to it
Don't cram for tests
Strive for understanding of concepts and processes

Session I

Chromosome Mechanics: How Genes Get Where They Are Supposed to Go

Before starting this session, study the following concepts and processes by reading the appropriate chapters in your text and studying your class notes:

> *mitosis: prophase, metaphase, anaphase, telophase*
> *meiosis: I, II*
> *haploid, diploid*
> *n, 2n, 3n*
> *interphase: G1, G2, S*
> *chromosome, chromatid*

Concepts/Processes	Level(s)	Relevant Question(s)	Page(s)
Cell cycle, DNA content, *n, 2n*	1, 1, 4	1, 2, 6	2, 4, 16
Gametogenesis	1, 3	2, 7	4, 18
3n, chromosome morphology	2, 2	3, 4	7, 9
Mitosis, meiosis, terminology	2, 3, 4	4, 5, 6	9, 12, 16
Nondisjunction, meiotic, mitotic	3	5	12
Anaphase configurations	4	6	16
Hybridization	1, 3	2, 7	4, 18

In a diploid organism (humans, for example) with a chromosome number of 46 ($2n = 46$) and a G1 nuclear DNA content of 13 picograms, what is the haploid number?

During metaphase of mitosis, how many chromatids are present in each somatic cell?

How many haploid sets of chromosomes are present in each cell?

What is the nuclear DNA content of a G2 cell? At metaphase, what is the expected cellular DNA content?

Concepts/Processes in Question 1: Fundamental to understanding genetics is a thorough understanding of **cell cycles** and **chromosome mechanics**. Terms such as **diploid**, **haploid**, **interphase**, **metaphase**, **chromosome**, and **chromatid** and symbols such as *n*, *2n*, **G1**, and **G2** must all be functionally and structurally related.

Analysis of Question 1:

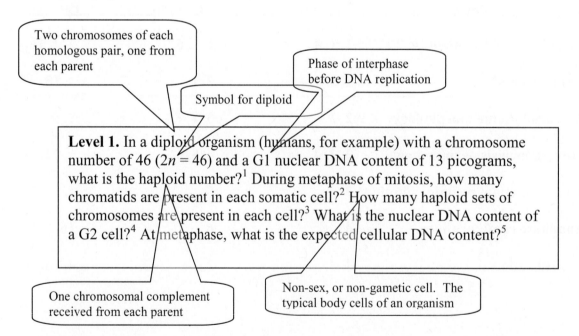

Two chromosomes of each homologous pair, one from each parent

Phase of interphase before DNA replication

Symbol for diploid

Level 1. In a diploid organism (humans, for example) with a chromosome number of 46 ($2n = 46$) and a G1 nuclear DNA content of 13 picograms, what is the haploid number?[1] During metaphase of mitosis, how many chromatids are present in each somatic cell?[2] How many haploid sets of chromosomes are present in each cell?[3] What is the nuclear DNA content of a G2 cell?[4] At metaphase, what is the expected cellular DNA content?[5]

One chromosomal complement received from each parent

Non-sex, or non-gametic cell. The typical body cells of an organism

Sentence 1 and answer: The diploid chromosome number represents all the chromosomes arriving from both parents during fertilization (haploid + haploid = diploid, or $n + n = 2n$). If the diploid chromosome number in an organism is known, the haploid chromosome number will be one half the diploid number; in this case 23 ($n = 23$).

Sentence 2 and answer: The metaphase stage of mitosis is characterized by the alignment of the replicated chromosomes equidistant and at the central plane between the two spindle poles of the cell. Since each chromosome has duplicated its DNA during the S phase of interphase, each chromosome should contain two chromatids, as shown below. Therefore, if there are 46 chromosomes in each cell, at metaphase, there should be 2 X 46 or 92 chromatids.

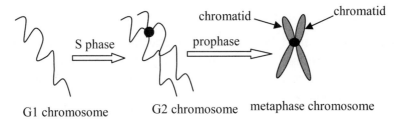

Sentence 3 and answer: Each parent contributes a haploid set ($n = 23$ chromosomes in this case) to the zygote (fertilized egg). Since the organism is diploid, there would be two haploid sets of chromosomes in a $2n$ cell. There would be 23 pairs of chromosomes, but only two haploid sets of chromosomes.

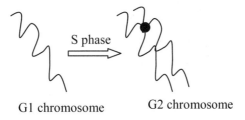

Sentence 4 and answer: Given that each G1 cell contains 13 picograms of DNA in its nucleus and that DNA replication occurs in the S phase leading to the G2 phase, there would be twice as much DNA (26 picograms) in a G2 cell compared with a G1 cell.

G1 chromosome   G2 chromosome

Sentence 5 and answer: Since a metaphase chromosome is a folded and condensed G2 chromosome without addition or subtraction of DNA, a metaphase chromosome would contain the same amount of DNA (26 picograms) as a G2 chromosome.

It is estimated that hookworms infect an estimated 740 million people worldwide. Of the 25,000 or so identified species of related worms, *Parascaris equorum* is of particular interest because it has only two chromosomes as its complete diploid complement.

(a) How many haploid sets of chromosomes would each somatic cell of *Parascaris* have? _____

(b) Assume that both chromosomes of *Parascaris* are metacentric (centromere in the middle). Sketch below the appropriate chromosomal arrangement for each cell type: Primary spermatocyte (metaphase I), primary oocyte (metaphase I), first polar body, secondary oocyte, mitotic metaphase.

Primary spermatocyte (metaphase I)

Primary oocyte (metaphase I)

First polar body

Secondary oocyte

Mitotic metaphase

Concepts/Processes in Question 2: This question requires an understanding of two critical terms, **diploid** and **haploid**. In addition, it asks for a depiction of chromosomes at critical stages of **mitosis** and **gametogenesis**. **Chromosome morphology** (metacentric) is introduced.

Analysis of Question 2:

A haploid set consists of the contribution from each parent

$2n = 2$ and $n = 1$

Level 1. It is estimated that hookworms infect an estimated 740 million people worldwide. Of the 25,000 or so identified species of related worms, one, *Parascaris equorum* is of particular interest because it has only two chromosomes as its complete diploid complement.[1] (a) How many haploid sets of chromosomes would each somatic cell of *Parascaris* have?[2] (b) Assume that both chromosomes of *Parascaris* are metacentric.[3] Sketch below the appropriate chromosomal arrangement for each cell type: Primary spermatocyte (metaphase I), primary oocyte (metaphase I), first polar body, secondary oocyte, mitotic metaphase.[4]

A metacentric chromosome has its centromere in the middle of its length

Sentence 1: Some background on the organism provides an interesting setting for this question; two chromosomes as the entire chromosomal complement. Therefore $2n = 2$ and $n = 1$.

Sentence 2 and answer (a): A haploid set is the chromosomal complement provided by one parent. Since two parents contribute to the zygote, and all somatic daughter cells have the same chromosomal content, there would be two haploid sets.

Sentence 3: There are four major classifications of chromosome structure depending on the position of the centromere relative to the chromosomal arms as shown below:

metacentric   *submetacentric*   *acrocentric*   *telocentric*

Sentence 4 and answer (b): Primary spermatocyte (metaphase I): because there are no sex differences for chromosomes mentioned, consider that at metaphase I (primary spermatocyte), the homologous chromosomes pair up at the metaphase plate.

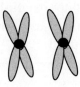

For a primary oocyte (metaphase I), the same configuration should occur.

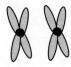

Since a first polar body and secondary oocyte have the same chromosomal constitution, each arising from separation of the homologous chromosomes, the following dyad should exist in each.

A mitotic metaphase has the $2n$ chromosomal number just as the primary oocyte and spermatocyte; however, generally, the chromosomes do not pair up. Therefore, a mitotic metaphase should have the following chromosomal configuration.

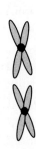

Assume that the typical diploid chromosome content of an organism is four chromosomes, two large and two small ($2n = 4$). Of the following figures, which represents a $3n$ metaphase chromosomal complement?

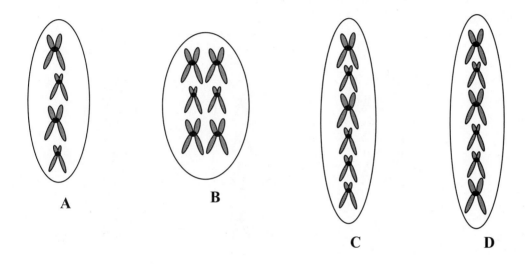

A   B   C   D

Assuming a DNA content of 12 picograms in each diploid G1 nucleus, what would be the expected metaphase DNA content of the $3n$ cell?

Concepts/Processes in Question 3: This problem requires an understanding of *n*, **2n**, and **3n** in terms of **chromosome complements for both mitosis and meiosis**. It also requires an adjustment in DNA content from G1 to metaphase as well as from $2n$ to $3n$. Careful inspection of **chromosome morphology** is also required.

We should now be looking for six chromosomes, three each of two types of chromosomes

Level 2. Assume that the typical diploid chromosome content of an organism is four chromosomes, two large and two small $(2n = 4)$.[1] Of the following figures, which represents a $3n$ metaphase chromosomal complement?[2] Assuming a DNA content of 12 picograms in each diploid G1 nucleus, what would be the expected metaphase DNA content of the $3n$ cell?[3]

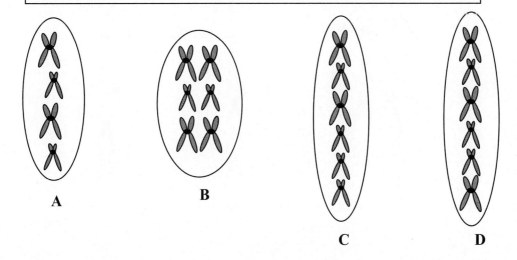

A   B   C   D

Sentence 1: Since we are talking about a typical diploid cell having four chromosomes, we would expect two homologous pairs of chromosomes. Notice that in figure "A" there are four chromosomes with two large chromosomes and two smaller chromosomes. Therefore, figure "A" illustrates an expected $2n$ chromosomal complement.

Sentence 2 and answer: Given the information from Sentence 1, for a $3n$ cell we should be looking for a cell with six chromosomes, but with three representatives for each type of chromosome. We have two types of chromosomes present, large and small. Figure "D" is the only one with three large and three small chromosomes. Notice in figure "B" there are four large and two small, while in figure "C" there are four small and two large. In addition, chromosomes appear to be paired in figure "B," which would not be expected of mitotic chromosomes at metaphase. Figure "D" provides the correct answer.

Sentence 3 and answer: If a G1 nucleus of a $2n$ cell contains 12 picograms of DNA, a G1 nucleus of a $3n$ cell should contain 18 picograms of DNA. Since DNA content doubles during the S phase, there should be 36 picograms of DNA in a metaphase $3n$ cell.

Question 4: Level 2

Consider an organism with a diploid chromosome number of 8.

(a) How many chromatids should be present at mitotic metaphase?

(b) How many tetrads are present in a metaphase I cell of meiosis?

(c) How many dyads are present in a meiotic metaphase II cell?

(d) How many monads are expected in the cells resulting from the completion of meiosis II?

(e) How many different kinds of gametes (assume no crossing over) would be expected as a result of independent assortment of chromosomes during meiosis?

Concepts/Processes in Question 4: This question gathers a number of important concepts and processes that occur during **mitosis** and **meiosis**. It addresses **chromatid** and **chromosome** structure during mitosis and meiosis as well as the behavior of such elements. In addition, important terms used to describe mitotic and meiotic events are presented (**tetrad, dyad, monad, independent assortment**).

> Dyads will be present after the first meiotic division

> Looking for the number of synapsed chromosome pairs

Level 2: Consider an organism with a diploid chromosome number of 8. (a) How many chromatids should be present at mitotic metaphase?[2] (b) How many tetrads are present in a metaphase I cell of meiosis?[3] (c) How many dyads are present in a meiotic metaphase II cell?[4] (d) How many monads are expected in the cells resulting from the completion of meiosis II?[5] (e) How many different kinds of gametes (assume no crossing over) would be expected as a result of independent assortment of chromosomes during meiosis?[6]

> Monads will be present after the second meiotic division

> Answer will be an integer based on the independent assortment of homologous chromosomes at meiosis I

Sentence 1: There are eight chromosomes in the total genome, so there should be four homologous chromosome pairs ($2n = 8$).

Sentence 2 and answer (a): Since each chromosome has duplicated during the S phase of interphase, each chromosome should contain two chromatids, as shown below. Therefore, if there are eight chromosomes in each cell, at metaphase, there should be 2 X 8 or 16 chromatids.

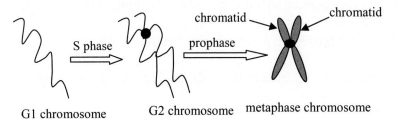

G1 chromosome   G2 chromosome   metaphase chromosome

Sentence 3 and answer (b): At the metaphase I stage of meiosis, homologous chromosomes typically synapse to form tetrads. As illustrated below, a cell that is $2n = 8$ should have four tetrads at the metaphase I stage.

Tetrad: four chromatids, two homologous chromosomes

Sentence 4 and answer (c): At meiosis I, homologous chromosomes go to opposite poles. The resulting dyads make up the cell's genome after meiosis I is completed. So each metaphase II cell should contain four dyads in each daughter cell, as illustrated below:

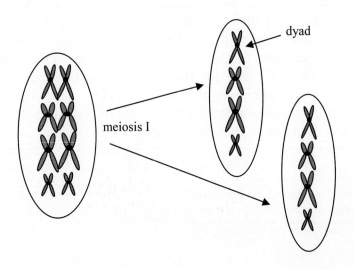

meiosis I

dyad

Sentence 5 and answer (d): As meiosis II is completed, there should be four monads in each of the daughter cells, as illustrated below:

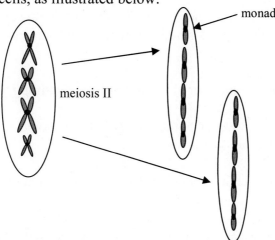

Sentence 6 and answer (e): Nonhomologous chromosomes align independently of each other at metaphase I. Therefore, with four homologous pairs of chromosomes ($2n = 8$) and each homolog separating independently of nonhomologs, there would be 2 X 2 X 2 X 2 = 16 different kinds of gametes. The formula, 2^n is often used to determine the number of different chromosomal combinations, where "n" is the number of chromosome pairs.

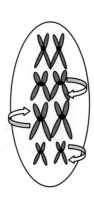

Question 5: Level 3

Assume that a diploid cell contains three homologous pairs of chromosomes designated as A_m, A_p, B_m, B_p, C_m, and C_p, where "m" stands for maternal origin and "p" stands for paternal origin.

(a) What is the $2n$ chromosome number in the individual containing this cell?

(b) Using the symbols given above, state the possible chromosomal composition of daughter cells of this cell following mitosis.

(c) State the possible chromosomal composition of the daughter cells following meiosis I.

(d) Assuming mitotic nondisjunction for the A_m chromosome, state the possible chromosomal composition of the daughter cells following mitosis.

(e) Assuming nondisjunction of the A_m chromosome at the first meiotic division, state the possible chromosomal composition of the daughter cells.

(f) Assuming normal disjunction at meiosis I, state the possible chromosomal composition of the daughter cells following nondisjunction of the A_m chromosome at meiosis II.

Concepts/Processes in Question 5: There are two components to this question that increase its level of difficulty over the previous questions in this session. First, chromosomes are represented by **abstract symbols** (A_p, B_m, etc.) rather than sketched and, second, important outcomes of **nondisjunction** are introduced for **mitosis, meiosis I,** and **meiosis II**.

Analysis of Question 5:

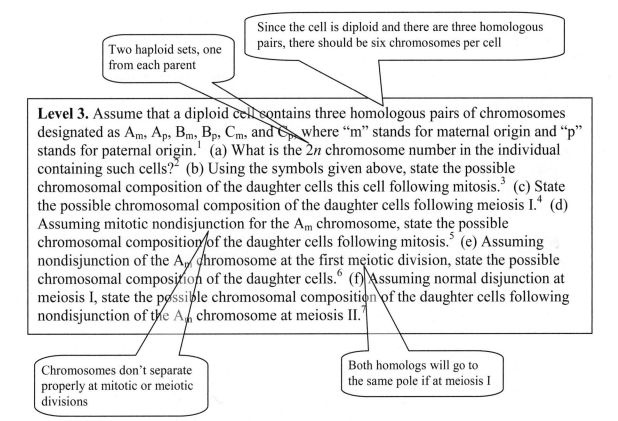

Two haploid sets, one from each parent

Since the cell is diploid and there are three homologous pairs, there should be six chromosomes per cell

Level 3. Assume that a diploid cell contains three homologous pairs of chromosomes designated as A_m, A_p, B_m, B_p, C_m, and C_p, where "m" stands for maternal origin and "p" stands for paternal origin.[1] (a) What is the $2n$ chromosome number in the individual containing such cells?[2] (b) Using the symbols given above, state the possible chromosomal composition of the daughter cells this cell following mitosis.[3] (c) State the possible chromosomal composition of the daughter cells following meiosis I.[4] (d) Assuming mitotic nondisjunction for the A_m chromosome, state the possible chromosomal composition of the daughter cells following mitosis.[5] (e) Assuming nondisjunction of the A_p chromosome at the first meiotic division, state the possible chromosomal composition of the daughter cells.[6] (f) Assuming normal disjunction at meiosis I, state the possible chromosomal composition of the daughter cells following nondisjunction of the A_m chromosome at meiosis II.[7]

Chromosomes don't separate properly at mitotic or meiotic divisions

Both homologs will go to the same pole if at meiosis I

Sentence 1: The conditions are quite clear here in that there will be six chromosomes total per cell and the homologous chromosomes will be symbolized as A, B, and C, with maternal and paternal chromosomes identified as shown below. Note that there can be a variety of ways of aligning the maternal and paternal pairs. As long as the chromosomes that look alike in the figure are identified by the same letter (A, B, or C), the labeling is valid.

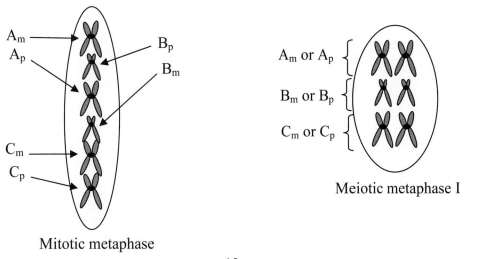

A_m

A_p

B_p

B_m

C_m

C_p

Mitotic metaphase

A_m or A_p

B_m or B_p

C_m or C_p

Meiotic metaphase I

Sentence 2 and answer (a): Given that there are three homolgous pairs of chromosomes, and the organism is diploid (see sentence 1), the *2n* complement must be six chromosomes.

Sentence 3 and answer (b): The question asks for the normal products of mitosis using the "letter" symbolism. Therefore, if you separate the sister chromatids to the daughter cells, each daughter should have the same chromosome composition as the parent cell: A_m, A_p, B_m, B_p, C_m, C_p.

Sentence 4 and answer (c): The figure above (meiotic metaphase I) shows that if one separates the homologous chromosomes as one typically does during anaphase I, each daughter cell should have the following combination of chromosomes: A_m or A_p, B_m or B_p, C_m or C_p --- in other words, three chromosomes, one from each homologous pair in any combination.

Sentence 5 and answer (d): Given nondisjunction of the A_m chromosome during mitosis, one would expect $2n + 1$ and $2n - 1$ for chromosome numbers in the daughter cells.

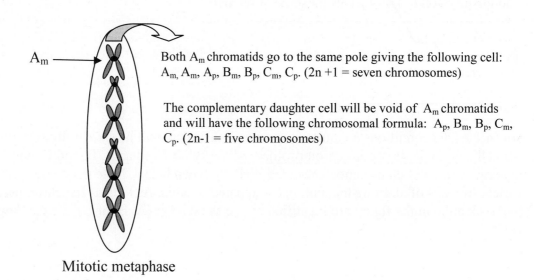

A_m

Both A_m chromatids go to the same pole giving the following cell: A_m, A_m, A_p, B_m, B_p, C_m, C_p. ($2n + 1$ = seven chromosomes)

The complementary daughter cell will be void of A_m chromatids and will have the following chromosomal formula: A_p, B_m, B_p, C_m, C_p. ($2n-1$ = five chromosomes)

Mitotic metaphase

Sentence 6 and answer (e): If nondisjunction occurs at meiosis I for the A_m chromosome, one would expect the daughter cells to have the chromosomal formula: $n-1$, and $n+1$, as shown in the figure below:

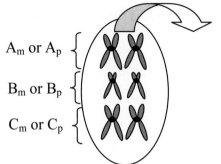

A_m or A_p

B_m or B_p

C_m or C_p

Meiotic metaphase I

If the A_m chromosome goes to the same pole as the A_p chromosome at anaphase I, the following cell will result: A_m, A_p, B_m or B_p, C_m or C_p. ($n+1$ = four chromosomes)

The complementary daughter cell would be void of an A chromosome and have the following formula: B_m or B_p, C_m or C_p ($n-1$ = two chromosomes)

Sentence 7 and answer (f): If nondisjunction occurs at anaphase of meiosis II for the A_m chromosome, sister chromatids will go to the same daughter cell and the complementary cell will be void of an A_m chromosome. The daughter cell receiving both Am chromatids will have a $n+1$ chromosomal formula and have 4 chromosomes. The complementary cell (not receiving either of the A_m chromatids) will have the $n-1$ chromosomal formula and have two chromosomes.

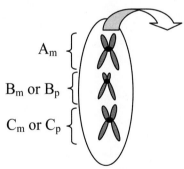

A_m

B_m or B_p

C_m or C_p

Meiotic metaphase II

If both of the A_m chromatids go to the same pole at anaphase II, the following cell will result: A_m, A_m, B_m or B_p, C_m or C_p. ($n+1$ = four chromosomes)

The complementary cell, receiving neither of the Am chromatids will have the following chromosomal formula: B_m or B_p, C_m or C_p. ($n-1$ = two chromosomes)

Assume that the following cell is viewed under a microscope and all the chromosomal material is visible. Assume also that the chromosomes are telocentric (centromere at one end), $2n = 2$, and the DNA content of a G1 somatic cell in this organism is 10 picograms.

(a) What stage of cell division is represented here and what would be its DNA content?

(b) Would your answers change if the chromosomes were metacentric (centromere in the middle of the chromosome)?

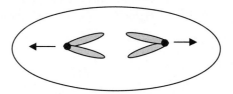

Concepts/Processes in Question 6: This question addresses relationships among **mitosis, meiosis, chromosome morphology**, and **DNA content**. Its proper solution requires a critical approach that integrates chromosome number and mitotic/meiotic events.

Analysis of Question 6:

This is an extremely important issue that will significantly influence the answer

Level 4. Assume that the following cell is viewed under a microscope and all the chromosomal material is visible.[1] Assume also that the chromosomes are telocentric (centromere at one end), $2n = 2$, and the DNA content of a G1 somatic cell in this organism is 10 picograms.[2] What stage of cell division is represented here and what would be its DNA content?[3] Would your answers change if the chromosomes were metacentric (centromere in the middle of the chromosome)?[4]

Completely changes the complexion of the problem

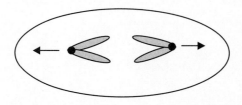

Sentence 1: The cell depicted is at anaphase as indicated by the centromeres being pulled to each pole. At this point it is impossible to determine whether the cell is in mitosis or meiosis; however, Sentence 2 will allow such a determination.

Sentence 2: The two most critical pieces of information in this sentence are that the chromosomes are telocentric and $2n = 2$. DNA content is also given, but in order to answer the question, the structure of the chromosome (telocentric) and chromosome number (two) are critical. Since the chromosomes are telocentric, the figure indicates that the chromatids have not separated, so these are the intact, duplicated chromosomes (with both chromatids) moving to the poles. Notice the two situations below:

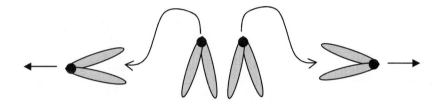

Anaphase I with homologous chromosomes moving to opposite poles

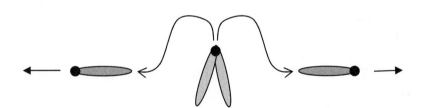

Anaphase of mitosis or anaphase II of meiosis with sister chromatids moving to opposite poles

Sentence 3 and answers: Since there are only two telocentric chromosomes in the cell and both of them are depicted in the figure, the figure shows homologous chromosomes moving to opposite poles. Therefore, the cell is in anaphase I of meiosis. With that being the case, there would be 2 X 10 picograms = 20 picograms of DNA in the cell.

Sentence 4 and answers: If $2n = 2$ and the chromosomes are metacentric, the picture changes entirely because the anaphase configuration would indicate that chromatids are moving to the opposite poles (see below). If that's the case, then the cell is in anaphase II of meiosis and there would be 10 picograms of DNA in this cell.

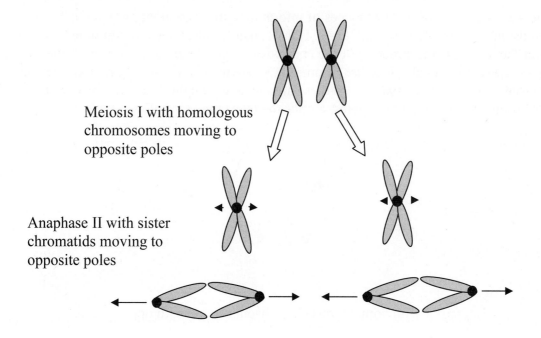

Meiosis I with homologous chromosomes moving to opposite poles

Anaphase II with sister chromatids moving to opposite poles

Question 7: Level 3

A species of wheat (*Triticum dicoccum*) has a chromosome number of 28, while a species of rye (*Secale cereale*) has a chromosome number of 14. Sterile hybrids can be produced by crossing these two plants.

(a) What would be the expected chromosome number in the somatic cells of the hybrids?
_____

(b) The G1 nuclear DNA content of *Triticum* is 5.5 picograms, and the G1 nuclear DNA content of *Secale* is 16.8 picograms. What would be the expected DNA content in a metaphase somatic cell of the hybrid?_____

Concepts/Processes in Question 7: This question requires an understanding of somatic and gametic chromosome numbers and, when gametes are combined, there may be an uneven chromosome number in a hybrid. Manipulation of DNA content is also required.

Analysis of Question 7:

2n = 28 and n = 14

2n = 14 and n = 7

Level 3. A species of wheat (*Triticum dicoccum*) has a chromosome number of 28, while a species of rye (*Secale cereale*) has a chromosome number of 14.[1] Sterile hybrids can be produced by crossing these two plants.[2] (a) What would be the expected chromosome number in the somatic cells of the hybrids?[3] The G1 nuclear DNA content of *Triticum* is 5.5 picograms, and the G1 nuclear DNA content of *Secale* is 16.8 picograms.[4] (b) What would be the expected DNA content in a metaphase somatic cell of the hybrid?[5]

Normal, nonsex cell, 2n body cells

Sentence 1: The chromosome numbers of the two species are presented, thereby giving information as to the gametic chromosome numbers ($2n = 28$ and $n = 14$; $2n = 14$ and $n = 7$).

Sentence 2: Hybridization among various plant species is common. Gametes with the expected chromosome numbers are formed and these gametes are combined.

Sentence 3 and answer (a): Since nothing unusual is expected, one can predict that the somatic cells of the hybrid would be the sum of the gametic chromosome numbers in the parents, namely, wheat ($n = 14$) and rye ($n = 7$). Therefore, the expected chromosome number in the somatic cells of the hybrid would be 21. Some students are bothered that the number is uneven. Remember, however, that the question is about somatic cells, where there is no need for homology or chromosome pairing, and that the hybrids are sterile (where, in gametogenesis, chromosome pairing is required).

Sentence 4: The DNA content in each G1 cell is given; from this the DNA content in all other cells can be computed.

Sentence 5 and answer (b): The G1 nuclear DNA content of *Triticum* is 5.5 picograms and the G1 nuclear DNA content of *Secale* is 16.8 picograms, and it is expected that each gamete would have half the DNA content of each G1 nucleus. Therefore, a gamete from *Triticum* would have 2.75 picograms of DNA while a gamete from *Secale* would have 8.4 picograms. Putting the two gametes together would produce a zygote with 11.15 picograms of DNA at G1. Considering that metaphase cells have 2X DNA compared with a G1 cell, there would be an expected 22.30 picograms of DNA in a metaphase cell of the hybrid.

Session II

Mendelian Genetic: The Heart of Transmission Genetics

Concepts/Processes	Level(s)	Relevant Question(s)	Page(s)
Conventional symbolism	1, 2	1, 2	21, 22
Monohybrid cross	1, 2	1. 2	21, 22
Dominant, recessive	1, 2	1, 2	21, 22
Heterozygous, homozygous	1, 2	1, 2	21, 22
Genotype, phenotype	1, 2	1, 2, 3	21, 22, 24
Probability	2-4	2, 3, 4, 5	22, 24, 25, 26
Product rule	1-4	2, 4, 5, 8, 9, 10, 11	22-26, 31-38
Binomial theorem	3	5	26
Pedigree analysis	2, 3, 4	6, 7, 8	27, 29, 31
Shortest path	4	8	31
Dihybrid cross	1	9	32
Testcross (backcross)	1	9	32
Independent assortment	1, 3	9, 11	32, 37
Fork-line method	1, 2, 3	9, 10, 11	32, 35, 37
Trihybrid cross	3	11	37
Complementing genotypes	4	12	39
Chromsomal basis of Mendelism	4	12	39

Question 1: Level 1

Albinism is caused by an autosomal allele that interferes with skin pigmentation in mammals. Two normally pigmented parents have an albino child. What is the probability that their next child will have albinism?

Components of your solution:

Diagram the cross using **conventional symbolism** that illustrates the **genotypes** and **phenotypes** of the parents and the *first* albino child:

What concept will you apply to determine the probability that the *next child* will have albinism?

Concepts/Processes in Question 1: There are three primary aspects to this problem. First, there is one gene pair involved, thereby specifying a **monohybrid cross.** Second, the allele for normal pigmentation is **completely dominant** to the allele giving albinism. Third, each union of gametes is independent of previous unions, and the **probability** of such unions can be determined. It is also important at this time to develop the use of conventional genetic symbolism.

Analysis of Question 1:

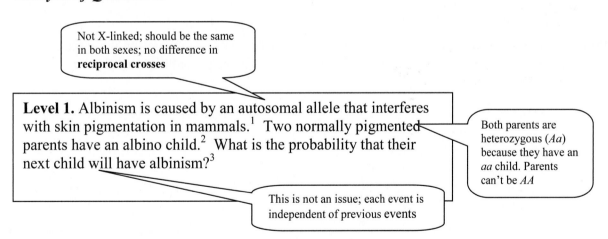

Not X-linked; should be the same in both sexes; no difference in **reciprocal crosses**

Level 1. Albinism is caused by an autosomal allele that interferes with skin pigmentation in mammals.[1] Two normally pigmented parents have an albino child.[2] What is the probability that their next child will have albinism?[3]

Both parents are heterozygous (*Aa*) because they have an *aa* child. Parents can't be *AA*

This is not an issue; each event is independent of previous events

Sentence 1: Since a single trait is referred to, it is likely that a **monohybrid** cross is described. The statement refers to mammals, so consider that all mammals could be involved with minor changes in the question (mice, rats, rabbits, etc.). Other vertebrates (birds, fish, amphibians, and reptiles) also can display albinism.

Sentence 2: If two normally pigmented parents have an albino child (*aa*), then each parent must be heterozygous (*Aa*). Albinism therefore involves a recessive allele so the **heterozygous** (*Aa*) individuals will be **phenotypically** identical to the **homozygous** (*AA*) individuals. See the dotted circle in this typical Punnett square of a monohybrid cross. If either parent were homozygous (*AA*), there would, under normal circumstances, be zero probability of making the *aa* combination.

Sentence 3 and answer: Probability simply refers to the chance of a given event out of all possible events. What is the chance of getting heads on a single coin flip? Since there are two alternatives (heads and tails), and you are asked about getting heads on a single flip, the probability is ½. Since there are four theoretical combinations of gametes in a simple monohybrid cross, and the question asks for the probability of getting the *aa* combination, the correct answer is ¼. You may be wondering whether the probability should change because the couple already had a child with albinism. Remember, a coin has no memory and each event (flip) is independent. Gametes have no memory, either!

Question 2: Level 2

Albinism is caused by an autosomal allele that interferes with skin pigmentation in mammals. Two normally pigmented parents have an albino girl. What is the probability that their next child will be a boy with albinism?

Concepts/Processes in Question 2: This question is essentially the same as Question 1; however, because the sex of the next child is requested, the **product rule** must be applied.

Analysis of Question 2:

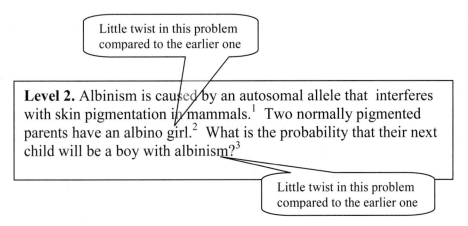

Sentence 1, same as Question 1: Since a single trait is referred to, it is likely that a **monohybrid** cross is described. The statement refers to mammals, so consider that all mammals could be involved with minor changes in the question (mice, rats, rabbits, etc.). Other vertebrates (birds, fish, amphibians, and reptiles) also can display albinism.

Sentence 2, same as Question 1, with a slight twist: If two normally pigmented parents have an albino child (*aa*), then each parent must be heterozygous (*Aa*). Albinism therefore involves a recessive allele so the **heterozygous** (*Aa*) individuals will be **phenotypically** identical to the **homozygous** (*AA*) individuals. See the dotted circle in this typical Punnett square of a monohybrid cross. If either parent were homozygous (*AA*), there would be no possibility of making the *aa* combination. The parents have a girl with albinism. There is no need to consider the fact that the first child is a girl. The sex of the first child is of no consequence to the answer.

Sentence 3 and answer: Notice that the sex of the second child is specified as boy. This requires the application of the **product rule,** according to which two or more events, if independent, can be multiplied to provide the probability of a final outcome. Since there is a ½ chance of getting a boy, the final probability is ¼ x ½ = 1/8.

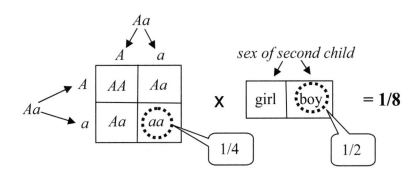

Albinism is caused by an autosomal allele that interferes with skin pigment in mammals. Two normally pigmented parents have an albino girl. What is the probability that their first male child will have albinism?

Concepts/Processes in Question 3: All the concepts/processes present in Question 1 are again addressed in Question 3 but this time a more thoughtful **application of probabilities** must be applied in order to arrive at the correct answer.

Analysis of Question 3:

Level 2. Albinism is caused by an autosomal allele that interferes with skin pigment in mammals.[1] Two normally pigmented parents have an albino girl.[2] What is the probability that their first male child will have albinism?[3]

Significant wording difference compared to the previous question

Sentences 1 and 2: If two normally pigmented parents have an albino child (*aa*), then each parent must be heterozygous (*Aa*). Albinism therefore involves a recessive allele so the **heterozygous** (*Aa*) individuals will be **phenotypically** identical to the **homozygous** (*AA*) individuals. See the dotted circle in this typical Punnett square of a monohybrid cross. If either parent were homozygous (*AA*), there would be no possibility of making the *aa* combination. The parents have a girl with albinism.

Sentence 3 and answer: There is a significant difference in wording in this question compared to the previous one. Notice that the sex of the second child is given, therefore, the probability of the child being male is 1/1 and the final probability become ¼ x 1/1 = ¼.

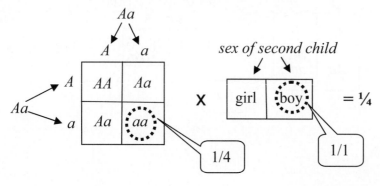

24

Albinism is caused by an autosomal allele that interferes with skin pigmentation in mammals. Two normally pigmented parents have an albino girl. What is the probability that their next three children will be normally pigmented?

Concepts/Processes in Question 4: All the concepts/processes present in Questions 1, 2, and 3 are again addressed in Question 4, except a slightly more extensive **application of the product rule** is applied.

Analysis of Question 4:

Level 2. Albinism is caused by an autosomal allele that interferes with skin pigmentation in mammals.[1] Two normally pigmented parents have an albino girl.[2] What is the probability that their next three children will be normally pigmented?[3]

Each child will have a ¾ chance of being normally pigmented

Sentences 1 and 2: If two normally pigmented parents have an albino child (*aa*), then each parent must be heterozygous (*Aa*). Albinism therefore involves a recessive allele so the **heterozygous** (*Aa*) individuals will be **phenotypically** identical to the **homozygous** (*AA*) individuals. If either parent were homozygous (*AA*), there would be no possibility of making the *aa* combination. The parents have a girl with albinism.

Sentence 3 and answer: Notice that the question is altered slightly in two ways. First, the question is requesting the probability of being normally pigmented and second, three additional children are born to these parents. The answer should be ¾ x ¾ x ¾ = 27/64.

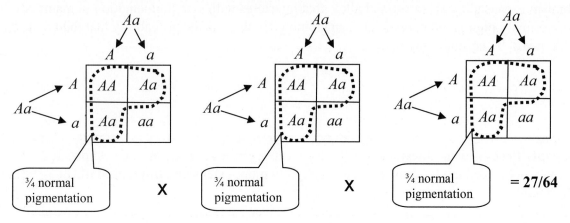

Albinism is caused by an autosomal allele that interferes with skin pigment in mammals. Two normally pigmented parents have an albino girl. What is the probability that three of their next five children will be normally pigmented?

Concepts/Processes in Question 5: This question involves all of the concepts/processes presented in the previous questions in this session; however, the problem involves determining the probability of a specified set of outcomes out of a larger number of potential outcomes. The **binomial theorem** is applied.

Analysis of Question 5:

Level 3. Albinism is caused by an autosomal recessive allele that interferes with skin pigment in mammals.[1] Two normally pigmented parents have an albino girl.[2] What is the probability that three of their next five children will be normally pigmented?[3]

A special case of the **binomial theorem** is involved here.

Sentences 1 and 2: If two normally pigmented parents have an albino child (*aa*), then each parent must be heterozygous (*Aa*). Albinism therefore involves a recessive allele so the **heterozygous** (*Aa*) individuals will be **phenotypically** identical to the **homozygous** (*AA*) individuals. See the dotted circle in this typical Punnett square of a monohybrid cross. If either parent were homozygous (*AA*), there would be no possibility of making the *aa* combination. The parents have a girl with albinism.

Sentence 3 and answer: This question requires that you calculate the probability of a specific set of outcomes (any combination in families of any size) from among a large number of possible events. One could compute an answer "the long way" by adding all the different possible combinations of events that would give two children with albinism and three normally pigmented children, however, this process would be laborious and error-prone. The following formula provides a shortcut.

$$p = \frac{n!}{s! \, t!} \, a^s \, b^t$$

n = total number of events (five in this case)
s = number of times outcome *a* happens (three in this case)
t = number of times outcome *b* happens (two in this case)
a = probability of being normally pigmented in this cross (3/4)
b = probability of being albino in this cross (1/4)

$$p = \frac{5!}{3! \, 2!} \, 3/4^3 \, 1/4^2$$

The overall probability (*p*) would be 270/1024 or about .26 (26%).

All these types of questions are handled in the same manner. Determine the total number of events (*n*), then how many times one outcome will occur (*s*). Determine how many times the alternative outcome will occur (*t*). Once you know the probability (*a*) of the "*s*" outcome and the probability (*b*) of outcome "*t*" you have all the components for the equation. Remember that "!" means factorial, for example: 5! = 5 x 4 x 3 x 2 x 1 = 120.

Question 6: Level 2

Given the following pedigree in which the shaded figures indicate the expression of a genetic condition, suggest a most likely pattern of inheritance.

Indicate the likely genotypes of each individual in the pedigree. What is the probability that the daughter (II-1) is heterozygous?

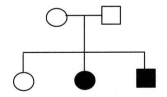

27

Concepts/Processes in Question 6: This problem provides a **pedigree** that is consistent with a simple **monohybrid** Mendelian trait with **complete dominance**.

Analysis of Question 6:

Level 2. Given the following pedigree in which the shaded figures indicate the expression of a genetic condition, suggest a most likely pattern of inheritance.[1] Indicate the likely genotypes of each individual in the pedigree.[2] What is the probability that the daughter (II-1) is **heterozygous**?[3]

Below are simple rules to help you decide the mode of inheritance when simple pedigrees are provided. While there are exceptions to the following statements, in general, the themes are consistent and will be applicable in a majority of the straightforward cases.

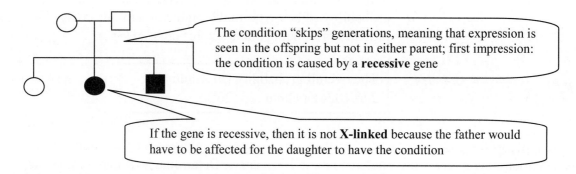

The condition "skips" generations, meaning that expression is seen in the offspring but not in either parent; first impression: the condition is caused by a **recessive** gene

If the gene is recessive, then it is not **X-linked** because the father would have to be affected for the daughter to have the condition

Sentence 1 and answer: Given the interpretations above, it is most likely that the condition is caused by a recessive allele that is **autosomal**, not X-linked.

Sentence 2 and answers:

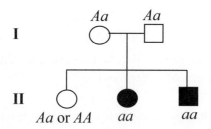

Sentence 3 and answer: Since individual II-1 does not have the condition, she is either *Aa* or *AA*. There is a 2/3 chance that she is heterozygous. Examine the following figure.

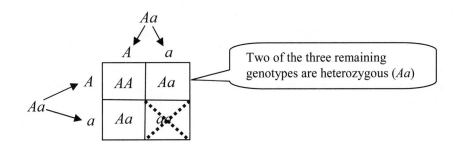

Two of the three remaining genotypes are heterozygous (*Aa*)

Question 7: Level 3

Given the following pedigree in which the shaded figures indicate the expression of a genetic condition, suggest a pattern(s) of inheritance that is(are) consistent with the data given. Assume that the condition is caused by an extremely rare allele.

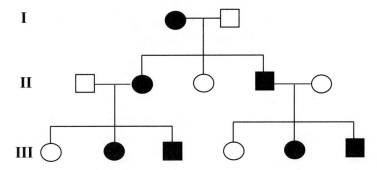

Concepts/Processes in Question 7: The pedigree is consistent with a simple **monohybrid** condition in which the trait is determined by **complete dominance**. Application of the **"rare gene"** component adds support for the complete dominance conclusion.

Analysis of Question 7:

Level 3. Given the following pedigree in which shaded figures indicate the expression of a genetic condition, suggest a pattern(s) of inheritance that is(are) consistent with the data given.[1] Assume that the condition is caused by an extremely rare allele.[2]

Suggestion is that there may be more than one consistent pattern, but multiple interpretations are not guaranteed

Gene is probably confined to the family and will not be introduced by outside individuals

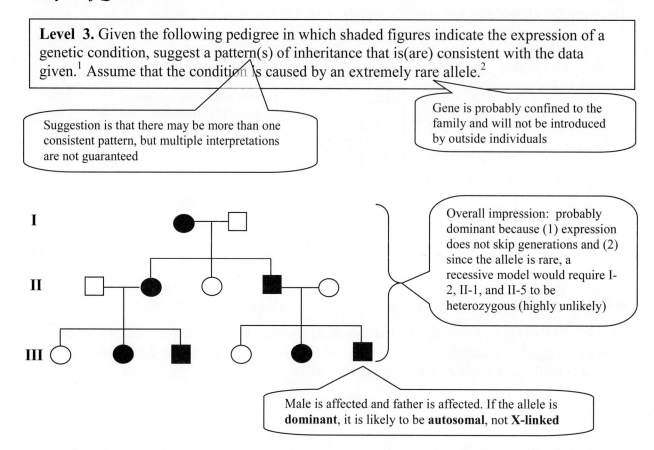

Overall impression: probably dominant because (1) expression does not skip generations and (2) since the allele is rare, a recessive model would require I-2, II-1, and II-5 to be heterozygous (highly unlikely)

Male is affected and father is affected. If the allele is **dominant**, it is likely to be **autosomal**, not **X-linked**

Sentences 1 and 2, and answer: Because the allele is rare, and therefore highly unlikely to be introduced from outside the immediate blood line, and no generations are skipped, a dominant gene is suspected. The fact that the III-6 male expresses the trait and that his mother does not, indicates that the gene is not X-linked because males inherit their X chromosomes from their mothers. So the pedigree is consistent with a dominant, autosomal allele.

Assume that a particular phenotype is caused by an autosomal recessive allele. John has a brother with the phenotype. Jane has a sister with the phenotype. No others in either family have the phenotype. John marries Jane and they decide to have a child. What is the probability that this child will be of normal phenotype?

Concepts/Processes in Question 8: While this problem involves a relatively simple **monohybrid analysis**, one must couple elementary **probability** with the **product rule**. In addition, the advantage of using the **shortest path** to the answer is also demonstrated.

Analysis of Question 8:

> Since John does not have the phenotype, he must have a 2/3 probability of being heterozygous . The same conclusion can be reached for Jane

> Looking for affected individuals to have the *aa* genotype

Level 4. Assume that a particular phenotype is caused by an autosomal recessive allele.[1] John has a brother with the phenotype.[2] Jane has a sister with the phenotype.[3] No others in either family have the phenotype.[4] John marries Jane and they decide to have a child.[5] What is the probability that this child will be of normal phenotype?[6]

> The question asks for the chances of being normally pigmented. It is much easier and more direct to first calculate the probability of being abnormal

> If John and Jane are heterozygous, they will have a ¼ chance of producing a child with the phenotype. But, we don't know whether John and/or Jane are heterozygous

Sentences 1 through 5: The best way to approach this type of question is to construct a pedigree that includes the pertinent information.

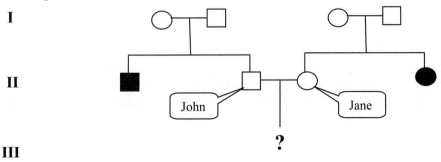

31

Sentence 6: The critical issue rests on the genotypes of John and Jane. If they are heterozygous, then the problem is simple. What are the probabilities that John and Jane are heterozygous? Examine the figure below and note that since John and Jane are of normal phenotype, they each have a 2/3 chance of being heterozygous. If they are heterozygous, the probability that they will produce the *aa* combination (affected phenotype) is ¼. Therefore, the overall probability of the "?" child being *aa* is 2/3 × 2/3 × 1/4 = 1/9. But the question is, "What is the probability that this child will be normal?" The best way to determine the probability of the normal phenotype is to subtract 1/9 from 1 to get 8/9. Because there are many "paths" to giving a normal phenotype, it is much easier and less error-prone to determine the probability of being abnormal (one path), and then subtract that probability from 1.

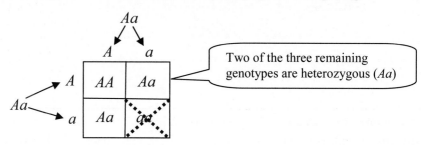

Two of the three remaining genotypes are heterozygous (*Aa*)

Question 9: Level 1

As Mendel found, the *full pod* condition is dominant to *constricted pods,* and the independently assorting *round seed* condition is dominant to *wrinkled seeds*. Crosses are made between full pod, round seed plants and constricted, wrinkled plants. The offspring all had the full and round phenotype. (a) When the F1 plants are crossed among themselves, what phenotypic ratio would be expected in the F2?

(b) If F1 plants are crossed with constricted, wrinkled plants, what would be the expected ratio in the offspring?

Concepts/Processes in Question 9: This question involves a straightforward **dihybrid cross** in part (a) and a **testcross (backcross)** in part (b). **Complete dominance** and **independent assortment** are stated conditions.

Analysis of Question 9:

> Two characteristics, pod shape and seed shape. Therefore, one would expect a dihybrid cross with two gene pairs

> Think about applying the symbols to the cross

Level 1: As Mendel found, the *full pod* condition is dominant to *constricted pods,* and the independently assorting *round seed* condition is dominant to *wrinkled seeds.*[1] Crosses are made between full pod, round seed plants and constricted, wrinkled plants.[2] The offspring all had the full and round phenotype.[3] (a) When the F1 plants are crossed among themselves, what phenotypic ratio would be expected in the F2?[4] (b) If F1 plants are crossed with constricted, wrinkled plants, what would be the expected ratio in the offspring?[5]

> Evidence that *full* and *round* are dominant to *constricted* and *wrinkled.*

> Pictured here are the two characteristics, pod shape and seed shape. Therefore one would expect a dihybrid cross with two gene pairs

> Pod shape

> Seed shape

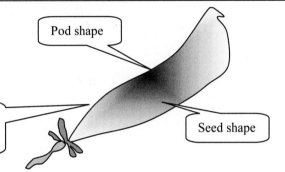

Sentence 1: This opening sentence identifies the genes involved, but more importantly it identifies the number of characteristics. Notice that there are two characteristics: pod shape and seed shape. With the knowledge of two characteristics involved in this cross, you can be fairly certain, although there are many exceptions (see Session III), that there are two gene pairs being described in this problem. This suggests a dihybrid cross. In addition, the dominance relationships are established, with *full pod* being dominant to *constricted pod* and *round seed* being dominant to *wrinkled seeds.*

Sentences 2 and 3: First, consider the cross as being in the "standard" format (*AABB* x *aabb*) but with different symbols, perhaps *CCWW* x *ccww.* You might ask "How do I know that the parental genotypes are homozygous?" There are two answers to this question: (1) some problems tell you to assume genotypes are homozygous unless given evidence to the contrary and (2) notice that the offspring all had the full and round phenotype. Had the full, round parent been heterozygous, there would have been some constricted and/or wrinkled plants in the F1.

So, at this point, here are the appropriate symbols:

Parents: *CCWW* x *ccww*

F1:   *CcWw*

Sentence 4 and answer (a): Because the F1s are *CcWw* and complete dominance and independent assortment are assured, the F2 would consist of the typical 9:3:3:1 phenotypic ratio. If you are not sure how this is determined, you must review the appropriate section in your text and lecture notes. If possible, try to identify the standard features of a typical (complete dominance and independent assortment) dihybrid cross without being dependent on filling out a 16-box Punnett square. Once you have done a 16-box Punnett square, you may identify shortcuts (fork-line method) that reduce the labor in doing straightforward problems of this type. Often, you can use the fork-line method because it is unlikely that you would be asked to fill in a 16-box Punnett square on an examination. In doing so, consider each gene locus separately, determine the phenotypes of each offspring, and then multiply the independent probabilities.

F1's are *CcWw,* so a cross of the F1's would be as follows:

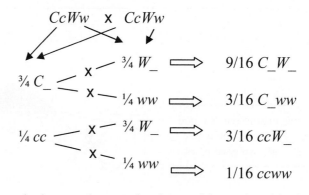

Sentence 5: Here again is a typical cross that can be done without the aid of a Punnett square. The cross is between the F1 (*CcWw*) and a *ccww* individual. This is the standard format of a testcross or backcross (the two terms mean essentially the same thing). Given complete dominance and independent assortment, a 1:1:1:1 phenotypic ratio will result. It is very important that you understand this because there are numerous applications that follow from this basic cross.

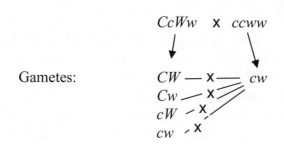

In a series of crosses involving pea plants that have round seeds and yellow cotyledons with pea plants that have wrinkled seeds and green cotyledons, the following ratios were observed in progeny. On the basis of these ratios, determine the genotypes of the parental plants for each set of crosses.

Parents	*Progeny*
(a) round, yellow **x** round, yellow	9/16 round, yellow
	3/16 round, green
Answer:	3/16 wrinkled, yellow
	1/16 wrinkled, green
(b) round, yellow **x** round, yellow	3/4 round, yellow
	1/4 wrinkled, yellow
Answer:	
(c) wrinkled, yellow **x** round, yellow	6/16 wrinkled, yellow
	2/16 wrinkled, green
Answer:	6/16 round, yellow
	2/16 round, green

Concepts/Processes in Question 10: This question is basically a reverse of Question 9 in that the **parental genotypes are requested** from offspring ratios. A simple **dihybrid** cross is involved with **complete dominance** and **independent assortment**.

Analysis of Question 10:

Level 2. In a series of crosses involving pea plants that have round seeds and yellow cotyledons with pea plants that have wrinkled seeds and green cotyledons, the following ratios were observed in progeny.[1] On the basis of these ratios, determine the genotypes of the parental plants for each set of crosses.[2]

Parents	*Progeny*
(a) round, yellow **x** round, yellow	9/16 round, yellow 3/16 round, green 3/16 wrinkled, yellow 1/16 wrinkled, green
(b) round, yellow **x** round, yellow	3/4 round, yellow 1/4 wrinkled, yellow
(c) wrinkled, yellow **x** round, yellow	6/16 wrinkled, yellow 2/16 wrinkled, green 6/16 round, yellow 2/16 round, green

---

Sentence 1: This sentence sets up the general parameters of the cross and gives the expectation of a typical dihybrid cross. At this point, you don't know which traits are dominant and which are recessive, nor do you know which phenotypes of the parents are represented by homozygous or heterozygous gene pairs.

Sentence 2 and answers: Before jumping into details, take a look at the general layout of the progeny ratios. Notice that for cross (a) the 9/16 class is round, yellow. This indicates that round is dominant to wrinkled and yellow is dominant to green. Given that dominance relationship, it's possible to quickly determine the parental genotypes for each of the crosses. Consider the following symbol sets: W = round, w = wrinkled; G = yellow, g = green.

Cross (a): Since the progeny fall into a typical 9:3:3:1 ratio, the parents must have both been heterozygous (*WwGg* **x** *WwGg*). If this is not obvious to you, then you must review the fundamentals in the previous problem and review this information in your text.

Cross (b): Notice first that all the offspring are yellow (*Gg* or *GG*) and the shape phenotype falls into a 3:1 ratio. Therefore, the parents must be one of the following: *WwGG* **x** *WwGG* or *WwGg* **x** *WwGG*.

Cross (c): Backing away from the details and examining each phenotype separately, notice that there is a 1:1 ratio (eight each) of round to wrinkled and a 3:1 ratio of yellow to green. This problem (and most like it) breaks down into two monohybrid crosses. So, since one of the parents is wrinkled yellow, it must be *ww* at the shape locus and *Gg* at the color locus (to give the 3:1 color ratio). The other parent is round yellow so it must be *Ww* to give the 1:1 shape ratio and *Gg* to give the 3:1 color ratio. Putting this information together gives the following genotypes for the parents: *wwGg* x *WwGg*.

Question 11: Level 3

Consider three independently assorting gene pairs *Aa*, *Bb*, and *Cc*. What is the probability (give a fraction) of obtaining each of the following genotypes from parents that are *AaBbCC* and *AaBBCc*?

      *AABbCC*_____   *aaBBCc*_____   *aabbCC*_____

Concepts/Processes in Question 11: This question involves a simple **trihybrid** crosss with **complete dominance** and **independent assortment.** It should be approached using the **fork-line method,** which applies the **product rule.**

Analysis of Question 11:

Level 3. Consider three independently assorting gene pairs *Aa*, *Bb*, and *Cc*.[1] What is the probability (give a fraction) of obtaining each of the following genotypes from parents that are *AaBbCC* and *AaBBCc*?[2]

      *AABbCC*_____   *aaBBCc*_____   *aabbCC*_____

Sentences 1 and 2, and answers: There are three loci described here, and since each is independently assorting, each can be handled separately, like three monohybrid crosses. Once the probability of obtaining each monohybrid result is determined, the product of the independent probabilities provides an overall probability. First, see if any of the outcomes are impossible. Notice that the last genotype *aabbCC* can't occur because *bb* can't result from a cross of *Bb* with *BB*. In some settings (timed examinations, etc.), this may be a useful shortcut.

For the first answer:

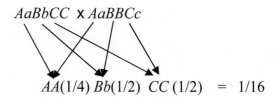

$$AA(1/4) \ Bb(1/2) \ CC(1/2) \ = \ 1/16$$

For the second answer:

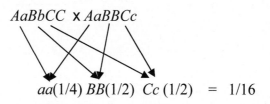

$$aa(1/4) \ BB(1/2) \ Cc(1/2) \ = \ 1/16$$

For the third answer:

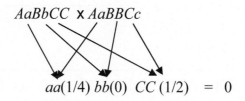

$$aa(1/4) \ bb(0) \ CC(1/2) \ = \ 0$$

Question 12: Level 4

Among several different types of albinism in humans is one form that is tyrosinase-negative (Type I on chromosome 11) and one that is tyrosinase-positive (Type II on chromosome 15). Evidence for their nonallelic nature was provided by a family in which two albino parents had four children (Trevor-Roper 1963).

(a) What pigmentation of the children would indicate that the two genes are nonallelic?

(b) Assuming that you could microscopically examine primary spermatocytes or primary oocytes of one of the children, what chromosomal and genetic constitution would such cells have? Sketch the chromosomes and their genetic makeup.

(c) Show how chromosomal behavior at anaphase I provides for independent assortment of the Type I and Type II loci for the child in part (b).

Concepts/Processes in Question 12: This problem requires a mastery of **genetic symbolism** and an understanding of the relationships among **genotypes**, **phenotypes**, and **chromosomal behavior during meiosis**. A **dihybrid** setup with **complementing genotypes** is involved.

Analysis of Question 12:

> Since the two loci are on different chromosomes, they are nonallelic. Picture gene loci on the two different chromosomes.

Level 4: Among several different types of albinism in humans is one form that is tyrosinase-negative (Type I on chromosome 11) and one that is tyrosinase-positive (Type II on chromosome 15).[1] Evidence for their nonallelic nature was provided by a family in which two albino parents had four children (Trevor-Roper 1963).[2] (a) What pigmentation of the children would indicate that the two genes are nonallelic?[3] (b) Assuming that you could microscopically examine primary spermatocytes or primary oocytes of one of the children, what chromosomal and genetic constitution would such cells have?[4] Sketch the chromosomes and their genetic makeup.[5] (c) Show how chromosomal behavior at anaphase I provides for independent assortment of the Type I and Type II loci for the child in part (b).[6]

Sentence 1: Because there are two different chromosomes involved, there must be two different gene loci giving the same phenotype: one produces tyrosinase, the other does not. Tyrosinase is one of the enzymes on the pathway to melanin, the skin pigment which, when lacking, produces albinism. In this problem, the enzymatic nature of the genetic lesions is irrelevant; however, the fact that one locus influences tyrosinase production and the other does not reinforces the chromosomal evidence that the two loci (Type I and Type II) are nonallelic.

Sentences 2 and 3, and answer (a): At this point set up the symbols for the cross. Once the symbols are in place, the answer to part (a) will be obvious. Since *evidence* for their nonallelic nature is given in this sentence, the two parents with albinism must each have the different gene loci:

Parent with Type I on chromosome 11: let *A* represent the functional allele and *a* represent the mutant allele.

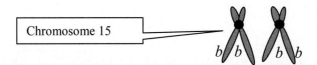

Parent with Type II on chromosome 15: let *B* represent the functional allele and *b* represent the mutant allele.

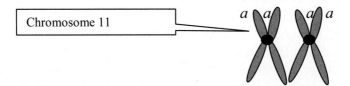

Accounting for the normal alleles for each parent would give the following genotypes and define the phenotype of the four children described in part (a) of the question.

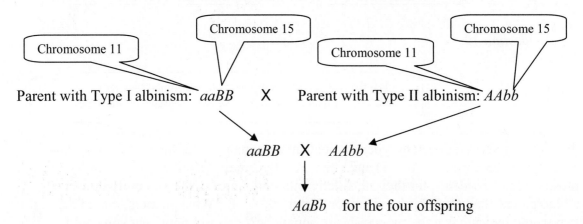

If the genes for Type I and Type II are nonallelic as indicated in the description of the problem and the above symbolism, the four children would have full pigmentation. The offspring would have normal alleles at each locus, giving a double heterozygote and full pigmentation. For the offspring to have albinism, they would have to have *aa*, *bb*, or *aabb* genotypes.

Sentences 4 and 5, answer (b): The question asks for an illustration of chromosomes in the **primary spermatocytes** and **oocytes** of the offspring. If you are uncertain about chromosome structure and alignment in primary spermatocytes/oocytes, be certain to review the appropriate sections of your text. Offspring have the genotype of *AaBb,* so the following configuration would be appropriate. Note, that there are two possible alignments of the nonhomologous chromosomes, as shown below.

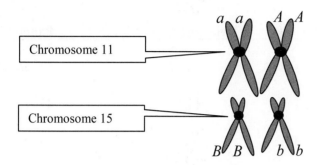

Sentence 6, and answer (c): Because the *A* (Type I) and *B* (Type II) loci are on nonhomologous chromosomes, two alignments (50% each) are possible, thereby accounting for independent assortment, that is, an equal frequency of each of the four gametes (*aB, Ab, AB, ab*).

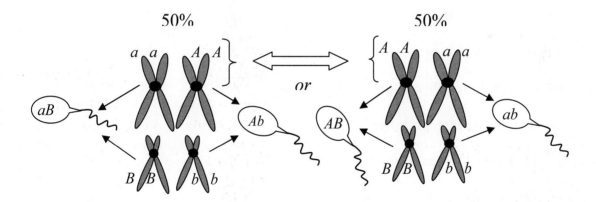

The next session **(Session III)** will ask you to apply what you have learned from Mendelian genetics to a variety of interesting, realistic, and often confusing extensions including allelic (incomplete dominance and codominance) and nonallelic interactions (epistasis, novel phenotypes, polygenic inheritance, lethality, etc.). Each extension requires a sound mastery of Mendelian genetics.

Session III

Applications and Extensions of Mendelian Genetics: Routine Genotypes but Varieties of Expressions

Concepts/Processes	Level(s)	Relevant Question(s)	Page(s)
Incomplete dominance	1, 3, 3	1, 3, 4	43, 46, 48
Codominance	2	2	45
Forked-line method, product law	3	4	48
Multiple alleles	3, 2	5, 6	50, 52
ABO blood groups, exclusion	2	6	52
Lethality, 2/3 ratio	2	7	54
Gene interaction, epistasis	2, 3	8, 9	57, 60
Epistasis and codominance	3	9	60
Gene interaction, novel phenotypes	3	10	62
Additive alleles, data interpretation	3	11	64
X-linked inheritance, probabilities	1	12	66
X-linked inheritance, nondisjunction	4	13	68

Question 1: Level 1

A cross was made between snapdragons with red and white flowers, and the resulting offspring were all pink. When the pink F1 snapdragons were crossed, the following offspring were produced: 125 red, 242 pink, and 121 white.

(a) What mode of inheritance is operating here?

(b) Assume that one of the pink F2 plants is crossed to a white plant. Of 400 offspring produced, what would be the expected numbers of red, pink, and white flowers?

Concepts/Processes in Question 1: There are four aspects to this question. First, one must recognize the **monohybrid** nature of the cross. Second, because the heterozygotes are recognizable (pink), **incomplete dominance** is likely. Third, **actual numbers** must be interpreted in terms of a **1:2:1,** ratio and last, a testcross ratio of **1:1** must be converted to actual numbers.

Analysis of Question 1:

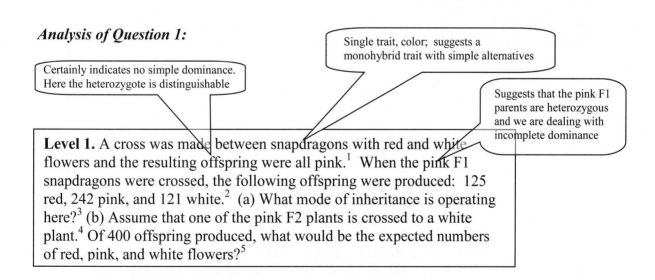

> Certainly indicates no simple dominance. Here the heterozygote is distinguishable

> Single trait, color; suggests a monohybrid trait with simple alternatives

> Suggests that the pink F1 parents are heterozygous and we are dealing with incomplete dominance

Level 1. A cross was made between snapdragons with red and white flowers and the resulting offspring were all pink.[1] When the pink F1 snapdragons were crossed, the following offspring were produced: 125 red, 242 pink, and 121 white.[2] (a) What mode of inheritance is operating here?[3] (b) Assume that one of the pink F2 plants is crossed to a white plant.[4] Of 400 offspring produced, what would be the expected numbers of red, pink, and white flowers?[5]

Sentence 1: At first glance, it appears that there is a single set of contrasting alleles with red and white genes being allelic. However, the offspring show up as pink, so another phenomenon must be involved. There is one likely possibility that should immediately come to mind when looking at this first sentence: incomplete dominance. With incomplete dominance, the heterozygote is generally intermediate in phenotype compared with either homozygote. We can assign symbols to help clarify the alleles involved. Typically, these symbols reflect the lack of dominance by both being similar, such as R^1, R^2 or W^1. The symbol set below will represent symbolically the alleles of the first cross.

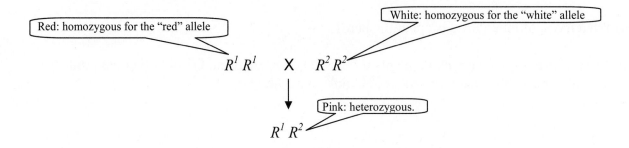

Sentences 2 and 3, and answer (a): The cross between two pink F1 snapdragons can be easily done without a Punnett square, however, one will be provided below for clarification in the event that you are more comfortable with that approach.

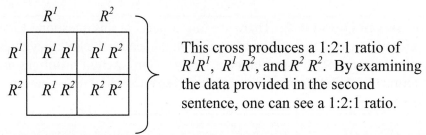

This cross produces a 1:2:1 ratio of R^1R^1, $R^1 R^2$, and $R^2 R^2$. By examining the data provided in the second sentence, one can see a 1:2:1 ratio.

(a) One main way to identify a case of *incomplete dominance* is to have the genotypic and phenotypic ratios be identical. At this point, all the information points to incomplete dominance as the mode of inheritance. There has been no change in the behavior of genes; they still obey Mendelian Laws. However, the phenotypes do not show dominance.

Sentences 4 and 5: The following symbols will illustrate a cross between a pink plant and a white plant.

$$R^1 R^2 \quad X \quad R^2 R^2$$
$$\downarrow$$
$$R^1 R^2 \quad and \quad R^2 R^2$$

Since there are only two kinds of offspring possible, and they would occur in equal frequencies (1:1), of 400 total produced, 200 of each (pink and white) should result.

Found on chromosome 4 in humans, two blood group alleles, L^M and L^N, are equally expressed in heterozygous individuals. Such heterozygous individuals are said to be in the MN blood group. Assume that a man and woman, both in the MN blood group, have a child.

(a) What is the probability that this child will be a girl and be in the MN blood group?

(b) What is the probability that the next two children born to this couple will be in the MM blood group?

Concepts/Processes in Question 2: There are two aspects to this problem. First, this is a **monohybrid** setup with **codominance**. Second, the **product law** applies in two different circumstances.

Analysis of Question 2:

> Might make the assumption that this is a monohybrid case involving codominance

> Blood group antigens tend to show codominance rather than incomplete dominance

> **Level 2.** Found on chromosome 4 in humans, two blood group alleles, L^M and L^N, are equally expressed in heterozygous individuals.[1] Such heterozygous individuals are in the MN blood group.[2] Assume that a man and woman, both in the MN blood group, have a child. (a) What is the probability that this child will be a girl and be in the MN blood group?[3] (b) What is the probability that the next two children born to this couple will be in the MM blood group?[4]

> For parts (a) and (b) apply information from Session II

Sentence 1: Since the first sentence refers to two alleles, this must be a monohybrid situation. There are also two clues that codominance is involved. The weaker of the clues is that these are blood group alleles. Often, blood group antigens are expressed in a codominant fashion. The second clue is stronger. Reference to "equally expressed in heterozygous individuals" strongly indicates that codominance is operating. If the condition is monohybrid, codominant, then the concepts learned from Question 1 in this session can directly apply.

Sentence 2: Notice a minor change in the reference to alleles (L^M and L^N) versus the MN blood group (phenotype). Such symbolism is common when referring to blood groups (e.g., $I^A I^B$ for
the AB blood group). From this sentence, one would assume that there are three genotypes and a corresponding three blood groups possible: $L^M L^M$ = MM, $L^M L^N$ = MN, and $L^N L^N$ = NN.

Sentence 3 and answer (a): By applying what was learned in Session II, this problem is straightforward. The probability of the first child being MN is 2/4 or 1/2 and the probability of being a girl is 1/2. Therefore, the overall probability of the first child being a girl and in the MN blood group is 1/4. For illustration purposes, a Punnett square is shown below; however, you might try doing such a problem without using a Punnett square.

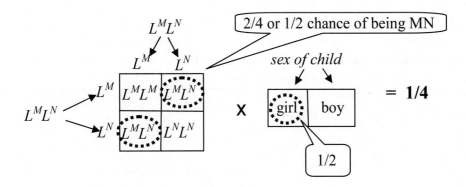

Sentence 4 and answer (b): When considering the above Punnett square, notice that the probability of a child being in the MM blood group is 1/4; therefore, the probability of the first two children being MM is 1/4 X 1/4 or 1/16.

Question 3: Level 3

Flower color in snapdragons is determined to some extent by a pair of alleles that show incomplete dominance: red, pink, and white with pink being the heterozygous class. Flower shape, mushroom versus normal, is determined by an independently assorting, single gene pair where *normal* is completely dominant to *mushroom*. Two pink snapdragons with normal flowers were crossed and produced, among 1600 total, 100 white, mushroom-flowered offspring.

What other types of offspring and how many of each are expected from this cross?

> **Concepts/Processes in Question 3:** This problem is a modification of a typical **dihybrid** cross with **incomplete dominance** of one allelic pair. The **forked-line** method of solution is preferred because it is quicker and, if applied correctly, less error-prone than dealing with a 16-box Punnett square. The problem also requires the **conversion from ratios to actual numbers**.

Analysis of Question 3:

> No linkage is involved so typical dihybrid ratios are expected

> Should produce a 1:2:1 ratio if pinks are crossed

> **Level 3.** Flower color in snapdragons is determined to some extent by a pair of alleles that show incomplete dominance: red, pink, and white, with pink being the heterozygous class.[1] Flower shape, mushroom versus normal, is determined by an independently assorting, single gene pair where *normal* is completely dominant to *mushroom*.[2] Two pink snapdragons with normal flowers were crossed and produced, among 1600 total, 100 white, mushroom-flowered offspring.[3] What other types of offspring and how many of each are expected from this cross?[4]

> Critical result here showing that both parents are heterozygotes

> Should produce a 3:1 ratio, if heterozygotes are crossed

Sentence 1: The pair of alleles in this problem show incomplete dominance, so if one crosses heterozygotes, there should be a 1:2:1 ratio (red, pink, white, respectively) in the offspring; see the Punnett squares dealing with flower color for Questions 1 and 2 above in this session.

Sentence 2: Flower shape, on the other hand, shows complete dominance, which would give a 3:1 ratio (normal, mushroom, respectively) in a cross of heterozygotes.

Sentence 3: Two pink, normal snapdragons are crossed, and finding white, mushroomed, offspring indicates that both parents were heterozygous (see below). This is a critical result because knowing the genotypes of the parents allows one to set up the cross and predict all the other offspring expected along with their numbers.

Sentence 4 and answer: The best way to approach this type of problem is through the forked-line method. Be certain to examine and practice the forked-line method illustrated in Session II, Question 9. As stated, there is independent assortment, so typical, albeit modified, Mendelian ratios are expected. Given that both parents are heterozygous, the cross is as shown below. By multiplying the individual probabilities, the final probabilities can be determined. From those final probabilities, multiplying by 1600 will give the expected numbers in each class. Let $R^1 R^2$ represent the pink-flowered genotype and *Mm* represent the heterozygous normal-shaped flowers.

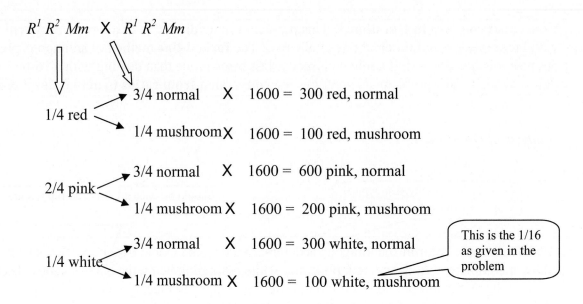

$R^1 R^2 Mm \times R^1 R^2 Mm$

1/4 red
- 3/4 normal X 1600 = 300 red, normal
- 1/4 mushroom X 1600 = 100 red, mushroom

2/4 pink
- 3/4 normal X 1600 = 600 pink, normal
- 1/4 mushroom X 1600 = 200 pink, mushroom

1/4 white
- 3/4 normal X 1600 = 300 white, normal
- 1/4 mushroom X 1600 = 100 white, mushroom

This is the 1/16 as given in the problem

Note: when doing a problem of this sort, always count up the offspring to be certain that they equal 100% of the total number of offspring.

Question 4: Level 3

Plumage in ducks is determined to some extent by a multiple allelic series of alleles named *restricted* (M^R = white on the wing fronts), *mallard* (M = wild type), and *dusky* (m^d = darker plumage). M^R is dominant to M, which is dominant to m^d.

(a) Can a mating between two mallard ducks produce any offspring with restricted plumage?

(b) A series of matings between two mallard ducks produced the following offspring: 34 mallard and 11 dusky ducks. What are the likely genotypes of the two mallard parents?

(c) Can a mating between two ducks with restricted plumage produce offspring with dusky plumage? Explain using diagrams of appropriate matings.

Concepts/Processes in Question 4: There are two main aspects to this problem. First, an understanding of **multiple alleles** and **dominance relationships** is required. Second, arriving at the correct genotypes of all individuals in crosses is essential to setting up and executing a solution.

Analysis of Question 4:

> Knowing the order of dominance is critical to developing correct answers

> Three alleles will show monohybrid type ratios --- because they are allelic

Level 3: Plumage in ducks is determined to some extent by a multiple allelic series of alleles named restricted (M^R = white on the wing fronts), mallard (M = wild type) and dusky (m^d = darker plumage).[1] M^R is dominant to M which, is dominant to m^d.[2] (a) Can a mating between two mallard ducks produce any offspring with restricted plumage?[3] (b) A series of matings between two mallard ducks produced the following offspring: 34 mallard and 11 dusky ducks.[4] What are the likely genotypes of the two mallard parents?[5] (c) Can a mating between two ducks with restricted plumage produce offspring with dusky plumage?[6] Explain using diagrams of appropriate matings.[7]

Sentence 1: Many surface characteristics of organisms are determined by multiple alleles in which major genes have alternative forms that directly influence expression. In mammals, various multiple allelic systems are common such as coat color in rabbits (full color, chinchilla, Himalayan, albino, etc.). In each case, because these genes are allelic, and because organisms are diploid, only two alleles can exist in an individual at one time. Therefore, monohybrid ratios are observed in crosses even though there may be multiple phenotypes possible. This may be a little confusing, but carefully examine your text and notes before completing this problem. Mastery of the genetics of multiple allelic systems will take a little extra effort.

Sentence 2: There are three alleles described: M^R is dominant to M, which is dominant to m^d, meaning that the following genotypic/phenotypic relationships exist.

Genotypes	*Phenotypes*
$M^R M^R$	restricted
$M^R M$	restricted
$M^R m^d$	restricted
$M M$	mallard
$M m^d$	mallard
$m^d m^d$	dusky

Sentence 3 and answer (a): Since mallard ducks can contain no M^R genes (otherwise they would be restricted --- see above table), there is no way, barring mutation, for two mallard ducks to produce a duck with restricted plumage.

49

Sentences 4 and 5, and answer (b): If 34 mallard and 11 dusky ducks are produced, this approximates a 3:1 ratio or a typical monohybrid cross between two heterozygotes. The cross to produce these results would be as follows:

$$M m^d \quad \text{X} \quad M m^d$$

$$\left. \begin{array}{l} M M \\ M m^d \\ M m^d \end{array} \right\} \text{mallard}$$

$$m^d m^d \quad \text{dusky}$$

Sentences 6 and 7, and answer (c): A cross between ducks with restricted plumage can produce offspring with dusky plumage, similar to answer (b).

$$M^R m^d \quad \text{X} \quad M^R m^d$$

$$\left. \begin{array}{l} M^R M^R \\ M^R m^d \\ M^R m^d \end{array} \right\} \text{restricted}$$

$$m^d m^d \quad \text{dusky}$$

Question 5: Level 3

A famous paternity battle arose when Joan Barry claimed that Charlie Chaplin, a star of silent movies, fathered her child. Blood typing in paternity cases was gaining widespread use in the 1990s, so Charlie's lawyers had all three blood typed. Joan had blood type A, Charlie had blood type O, and the daughter had blood type B. The jury in the case ruled that Charlie had fathered the child. Do you agree with this verdict?

Concepts/Processes in Question 5: This problem involves an application of the genetics of **multiple alleles** to a common marker system (**ABO blood types**) in humans. An understanding of **dominance**, **codominance**, and **recessiveness** is necessary.

Analysis of Question 5:

> The ABO blood types represent a classic case of multiple alleles because both complete dominance and codominance are illustrated

Level 3. A famous paternity battle arose when Joan Barry claimed that Charlie Chaplin, a star of silent movies, fathered her child.[1] Blood typing gaining was widespread use in the 1990s, so Charlie's lawyers had all three blood typed.[2] Joan had blood type A, Charlie had blood type O, and the daughter had blood type B?[3] The jury in the case ruled that Charlie had fathered the child.[4] Do you agree with this verdict?[5]

Sentences 1 and 2: Paternity can often be excluded under certain circumstances by the use of blood typing. Usually, the mother's link to a child is clear. However, if a child has an allele that matches the mother but another allele that doesn't match the suspected father, the male can be excluded from being the father. If the suspected father contains genes or alleles like those of the child (that could not come from the mother), the male is not excluded as being the father. It is important to note that not being excluded does not prove paternity. Another person with the same gene(s) or allele(s) as that male may be the father. Below is a table that indicates the three alleles (multiple alleles) related to this problem. Notice that because these genes are allelic, they can only occur two at a time in any one individual.

Genotypes	*Phenotypes (blood type)*
$I^A I^A$ or $I^A i$	**A**
$I^B I^B$ or $I^B i$	**B**
$I^A I^B$	**AB**
$i\,i$	**O**

Sentence 3: If Joan had blood type **A**, she would be $I^A I^A$ or $I^A i$. If Charlie had blood type **O**, he would be $i\,i$. The genotype of a **B** blood type child could be $I^B I^B$ or $I^B i$.

Sentence 4 and 5, and answer: Examining the information provided in Sentence 3, and comparing it to the chart above, shows that the child has an "unexplained" I^B allele. The mother must have contributed either the I^A or i allele and Charlie could only have contributed i to a child. Therefore, the genetics indicates that Charlie is not the father (he is excluded). Assuming no other rare events (mutation, chimerism, etc.), the jury must have made an error.

Question 6: Level 2

A long-studied strain of mice, *yellow*, has recently revealed an interesting relationship with obesity. In addition to being a dominant gene conferring yellow coat color, A^Y behaves as a recessive lethal. In terms of obesity, A^Y/a mice develop hyperleptinemia and leptin resistance with age. Below is a list containing the results of crosses involving the coat color alleles described above. In each case, provide the genotypes of the parents and explain the genetics of the system.

(a) wild coat   X   wild coat   = all wild fur

(b) yellow coat   X   yellow coat   = 2/3 yellow coat; 1/3 wild coat

(c) wild coat   X   yellow coat   = 1/2 yellow coat; 1/2 wild coat

---

Concepts/Processes in Question 6: Recognizing the **dual expression** of the A^Y allele (dominant yellow and **recessive lethal**) is essential to assigning the appropriate genotypes to parts (a), (b), and (c). Since A^Y behaves as a recessive lethal, it must be homozygous to be expressed. The **distortion of the typical 1:2:1** ratio results from the recessive lethal action of A^Y.

Analysis of Question 6:

> This gene has an interesting behavior with two components to its action: lethality and coat color

Level 2. A long-studied strain of mice, *yellow*, has recently revealed an interesting relationship with obesity.[1] In addition to being a dominant gene conferring yellow coat color, A^Y behaves as a recessive lethal.[2] In terms of obesity, A^Y/a mice develop hyperleptinemia and leptin resistance with age.[3] Below is a list containing the results of crosses involving the coat color alleles described above.[4] In each case, provide the genotypes of the parents and explain the genetics of the system.[5]

(a) wild coat   X   wild coat   = all wild fur
(b) yellow coat   X   yellow coat   = 2/3 yellow coat; 1/3 wild coat
(c) wild coat   X   yellow coat   = 1/2 yellow coat; 1/2 wild coat

Sentence 1: Since mice typically have a brownish coat, often called wild or agouti, the yellow coat color must be a genetic variant. At this point no information is given about the genetics of coat color.

Sentence 2: The meat of the problem rests in this sentence. The gene A^Y behaves in two ways: as a recessive in terms of lethality and as a dominant in terms of coat color. Therefore, the A^Y/A^Y combination must be lethal (dies), and the heterozygous condition A^Y/a must have the yellow coat phenotype. The a/a genotype must have the wild or agouti coat pattern.

Sentence 3: This sentence, while interesting, has no bearing on the problem.

Sentences 4 and 5, and answers: Taking the information as stated in the problem, the following solution emerges. The key here is that the A^Y/A^Y combination is lethal and not recovered in the offspring. This is seen in the data with the 2/3 progeny ratio. Generally, any time you see a 2/3 progeny ratio, suspect lethality.

(a) wild coat   X   wild coat   = all wild fur

      a/a X a/a = all a/a

(b) yellow coat X yellow coat = 2/3 yellow coat; 1/3 wild coat

     A^Y/a X A^Y/a = 1/4 A^Y/A^Y, 2/4 A^Y/a, 1/4 a/a

> This combination is lethal and because it is only expressed as a homozygote, it must act as a recessive

> Since ¼ of the offspring were lost to lethality, of the survivors, 2/3 would have the yellow phenotype because they have the A^Y gene. The remaining 1/3 would have wild coat colors

(c) wild coat X yellow coat = 1/2 yellow coat; 1/2 wild coat

    a/a X A^Y/a = 1/2 A^Y/a, 1/2 a/a

Question 7: Level 3

A long-studied strain of mice, *yellow*, has recently revealed an interesting relationship with obesity. In addition to being a dominant allele conferring yellow coat color, A^Y behaves as a recessive lethal. An unrelated and unlinked recessive gene, *cappuccino* (*cno*), produces, among other things, pale eyes when homozygous. Extending the information presented in Question 6 above, consider results from crosses between mice with yellow coat color and normal eyes and mice with agouti coats and cappuccino eyes.

(a) Diagram such a cross by presenting appropriate genotypes and phenotypes.

(b) If the yellow-bodied offspring from cross (a) are crossed to their yellow-bodied siblings, what would be the expected phenotypic ratio in the offspring?

Concepts/Processes in Question 7: This problem requires careful application of **appropriate symbolism** and **adjustment to lethality** that **distorts a 9:3:3:1** ratio (part b). Use of the **forked-line method** greatly facilitates a rapid and accurate solution.

Analysis of Question 7:

A second gene is mentioned, indicating at least a dihybrid cross

Level 3. A long-studied strain of mice, *yellow*, has recently revealed an interesting relationship with obesity.[1] In addition to being a dominant allele conferring yellow coat color, A^Y behaves as a recessive lethal.[2] An unrelated and unlinked recessive gene, *cappuccino* (*cno*), produces, among other things, pale eyes when homozygous.[3] Extending the information presented in Question 6 above, consider results from crosses between mice with yellow coat color and normal eyes and mice with agouti coats and cappuccino eyes.[4] (a) Diagram such a cross by presenting appropriate genotypes and phenotypes.[5] (b) If the yellow-bodied offspring from cross (a) are crossed to their yellow-bodied siblings, what would be the expected phenotypic ratio in the offspring?[6]

Since the yellow gene is lethal in the homozygous state, all yellow mice should be heterozygous

Mice with agouti coats will be homozygous and those with cappuccino eyes will be homozygous for the mutant gene

Sentence 1 (as in Question 6): Since mice typically have a brownish coat, often called wild or agouti, the yellow coat color must be a genetic variant. At this point no information is given about the genetics of coat color.

Sentence 2 (as in Question 6): The gene, A^Y, behaves in two ways: as a recessive in terms of lethality and as dominant in terms of coat color. Therefore, the A^Y/A^Y combination must be lethal (dies), and the heterozygous condition A^Y/a must have the yellow coat phenotype. The *a/a* genotype must have the wild or agouti coat pattern.

Sentence 3: The appearance of the *cappuccino* gene (*cno*) opens up a new dimension to the problem, giving it a dihybrid look with underlying dihybrid ratios. Since the *cno* gene is recessive, a pale-eyed mouse would be homozygous *cno/cno*.

Sentences 4 and 5, and answer (a): Below is appropriate symbolism for the cross described. When doing these types of problems, it is very important to account for all the alleles involved, regardless of whether they are the mutants or the wild type alleles of the mutants. Notice below that all genes are fully accounted for. Note: the semicolon is often used to symbolize genes on different chromosomes.

$A^Y/a;Cno/Cno$	X	$a/a;cno/cno$	=	1/2 $A^Y/a;Cno/cno$,	1/2 *a/a, Cno/cno*
yellow body		cappuccio eyes		yellow body	wild (agouti)

Sentence 6 and answer (b): Offspring from cross (a) will produce a modified dihybrid ratio because all the A^Y/A^Y individuals are lethal. Using the forked-line method rather than the Punnett square, the following describes the cross. Proceeding as discussed in Session II, deal with each allelic gene pair separately, then multiply each outcome for the final ratio. Since phenotypes are requested, only phenotypes are needed; however, genotypes are provided for clarity.

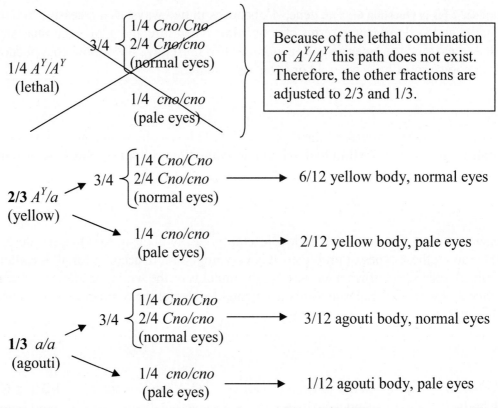

The resulting ratio becomes 6:2:3:1 because of the loss of the A^Y/A^Y path. Again, always add up the fractions in the progeny to be certain that all are accounted for. A total of 12/12 is needed in this case.

Coat color in mice is determined to some extent by two independently assorting but interacting gene loci. The dominant gene (*B*) at one locus allows a colorless precursor to form black pigment while its allele *b* inhibits pigment formation entirely and gives the albino phenotype when homozygous. The other locus, *A,* allows pigment to be deposited in the wild or agouti pattern. In the absence of *A* (i.e., when *aa* is the genotype), only the black pigment pattern occurs in the fur.

(a) From the information presented, sketch out the developmental pathway that leads to the wild or agouti coat pattern.

(b) Assume crosses are made between two fully heterozygous mice. What phenotypes would be expected and in what numbers if 160 offspring are produced?

(c) Again, assuming 160 offspring, what numbers in each phenotypic class would be expected in a series of matings involving *AaBb* and *aabb* mice?

Concepts/Processes in Question 8: This problem contains three major aspects. First, one must correctly interpret the phenotypes given in terms of possible and appropriate gene symbols. Second, one must relate the phenotypes to a **proposed pathway**. Third, it is possible to quickly arrive at correct answers if concepts surrounding **9:3:3:1** and **1:1:1:1** ratios are understood.

Analysis of Question 8:

"Interacting" typically suggests that the two gene pairs influence the same characteristic, coat color in this case

"Independently assorting" means that no linkage and typical Mendelian ratios (and their modifications) are expected

Level 2. Coat color in mice is determined to some extent by two independently assorting but interacting gene loci.[1] The dominant gene (*B*) at one locus allows a colorless precursor to form black pigment while its allele *b* inhibits pigment formation entirely and gives the albino phenotype when homozygous.[2] The other locus, *A,* allows pigment to be deposited in the wild or agouti pattern.[3] In the absence of *A* (i.e. when *aa* is the genotype) only the black pigment pattern occurs in the fur.[4] (a) From the information presented, sketch out the developmental pathway that leads to the wild or agouti coat pattern.[5] (b) Assume crosses are made between two fully heterozygous mice.[6] What phenotypes would be expected and in what numbers if 160 offspring are produced?[7] (c) Again assuming 160 offspring, what numbers in each phenotypic class would be expected in a series of matings involving *AaBb* and *aabb* mice?[8]

Sentence 1: The implication is that there are two loci in this problem, but there are probably more loci that relate to coat color determination. In fact, there are many such loci in mammals. The statement "independently assorting" signifies no linkage, and typical Mendelian genotypic ratios will apply. Because this is a problem dealing with epistasis, the Mendelian ratios will be modified at the phenotypic level. The statement that these are "interacting gene loci" signals that they probably influence the expression of one characteristic, in this case, coat color.

Sentence 2: The two loci described with locus *B* are involved in the following conversion:

$$\text{colorless precursor} \xrightarrow{\;\;BB\ or\ B\_\;\;} \text{black pigment}$$

When *B* is absent, e.g. *bb*, the pathway is blocked and no black pigment is deposited in the hair.

colorless precursor ⟶‖⟶ black pigment (albino) ✗

Sentences 3 and 4: When *A* (*A* or *A*_) is present, pigment is deposited in the wild-type or agouti pattern.

$$\text{black pigment} \xrightarrow{\;\;AA\ or\ A\_\;\;} \text{agouti pattern}$$

black pigment ⟶‖⟶ agouti pattern ✗ *aa*

Sentence 5 and answer (a): Combining the two above pathways into one yields the following pathway:

$$\text{colorless precursor} \xrightarrow{\;\;BB\ or\ B\_\;\;} \text{black pigment} \xrightarrow{\;\;AA\ or\ A\_\;\;} \text{agouti pattern}$$

Sentences 6 and 7, and answer (b): A cross between two fully heterozygous mice would be symbolized as shown below. This would be a typical dihybrid cross that would normally yield a 9:3:3:1 ratio if no gene interaction occurred. However, because of gene interaction, a modified phenotypic ratio will result, as shown below:

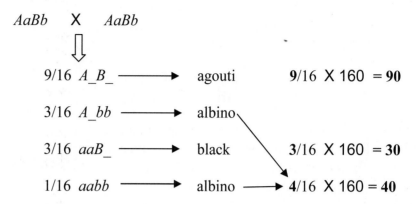

AaBb   X   *AaBb*

9/16 *A_B_* ——————→ agouti   9/16 X 160 = **90**

3/16 *A_bb* ——————→ albino

3/16 *aaB_* ——————→ black   3/16 X 160 = **30**

1/16 *aabb* ——————→ albino ——→ 4/16 X 160 = **40**

Notice that because two phenotypic classes (3/16 and 1/16) have the same phenotype, the phenotypic ratio is 9:3:4 rather than the typical dihybrid ratio of 9:3:3:1. Since the question asks for the actual numbers of offspring expected out of 160, multiplying each fraction by 160 provides the answers. In cases involving epistasis, one gene pair masks the expression of other nonallelic gene pairs. Here, because of *bb*, the expression of genes at the "*A*" locus is masked. There are many kinds of epistasis, and a student would do well to study from the text and lecture notes various aspects of epistasis in some detail.

Sentence 8 and answer (c): This section of the problem sets up a simple dihybrid backcross (or testcross) in that the double heterozygote is crossed to the fully recessive. The cross is therefore:

AaBb   X   *aabb*

1/4 *AaBb* ——————→ agouti   1/4 X 160 = **40**

1/4 *Aabb* ——————→ albino

1/4 *aaBb* ——————→ black   1/4 X 160 = **40**

1/4 *aabb* ——————→ albino ——→ 2/4 X 160 = **80**

Again, because of epistasis, two phenotypic classes have the same phenotype which gives a ratio of 1:1:2 and actual numbers, when multiplied by 160, of 40, 40, and 80.

Below is a partial pedigree of a family with individual ABO blood phenotypes.

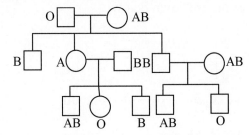

(a) Given these phenotypes, there is an apparent inconsistency. **Circle** the portion of the pedigree that identifies this inconsistency. Given that this problem involves epistasis, provide a genotype for the "inconsistent individual" that appropriately explains the apparent inconsistency.

(b) Next to the appropriate individuals, give the likely genotypes for the parents of this "inconsistent" individual such that the inconsistency is explained.

Concepts/Processes in Question 9: There are two main components in this problem: **multiple alleles** and **epistasis**. Successful solution requires an understanding of the interaction between the alleles that determine the **ABO blood groups** and those that are epistatic to those genes.

Analysis of Question 9

Recall the genetics of the ABO
blood types:

Genotypes	Phenotypes
$I^A I^A$ or $I^A i$	A
$I^B I^B$ or $I^B i$	B
$I^A I^B$	AB
$i\,i$	O

Level 3. Below is a partial pedigree of a family with individual ABO blood phenotypes.[1]

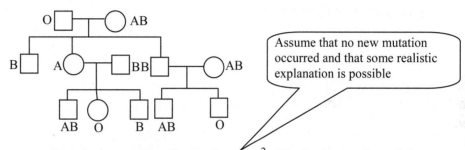

Assume that no new mutation
occurred and that some realistic
explanation is possible

(a) Given these phenotypes, there is an apparent inconsistency.[2] **Circle** the portion of the pedigree that identifies this inconsistency.[3] Given that this problem involves epistasis, provide a genotype for the "inconsistent individual" that appropriately explains the apparent inconsistency.[4] (b) Next to the appropriate individuals, give the likely genotypes for the parents of this "inconsistent" individual such that the inconsistency is explained.[5]

Sentences 1, 2, and 3: The pedigree is describing the ABO phenotypes of related individuals, and all components are consistent with expectations except for one, at the lower right. Since the parents are type B and AB, they must have the genotypes of $I^B i$ or $I^B I^B$ and $I^A I^B$, respectively. As such, it is impossible for them to produce an *ii* offspring under the narrow confines of the ABO alleles. Something else must account for the inconsistency.

Sentence 4 and answer (a): If the genotype of the "inconsistent" individual with blood type O was homozygous for the *FUT* allele, with a failed fucosyltransferas, there would be no H substance upon which function of the I^A and/or I^B alleles is dependent. In this case, there is no production of the A or B antigens. The exceptional individual with blood type O is really one of the following: $I^B i hh$, $I^A i\ hh$, $I^A I^B hh$, or $I^B I^B hh$. Note: this condition is a classic example of epistasis involving human blood types and is called the Bombay phenotype.

Sentence 5 and answer (b): The parents of the exceptional individual with blood type O must have each carried the *h* allele in the heterozygous state (*Hh*), because they were able to display the A and B antigens. Technically, they would have each had one functional *FUT1* gene.

Question 10: Level 3

The typical eye color of wild-type *Drosophila melanogaster*, the fruit fly, is a combination of red and brown pigments giving a dull, brick-colored red appearance. While a number of different genes influence eye color in *Drosophila*, two are the focus of this question.[2] The *brown* locus (bw^+, bw) on chromosome II influences the red pigment pathway, while the *scarlet* locus (st^+, st) influences the brown pigment pathway. Note: in *Drosophila*, the superscript "+" indicates wild-type alleles that are both dominant in these cases. In a cross between two doubly heterozygous flies, each having dull red eyes, the following eye colors resulted in the offspring: 96 dull red, 32 brown, 29 bright red, and 11 white. Provide an explanation for these results and explain why the term "novel phenotype" might apply.

Concepts/Processes in Question 10: This question requires an understanding of **novel phenotypes** applied to a typical **dihybrid cross**. To fully understand this problem, it would be helpful to know the biochemical underpinnings of **eye color formation in *Drosophila***.

Analysis of Question 10:

> Because the loci are on different chromosomes, they will show independent assortment; i.e., no linkage

> Think of blending red and brown pigments: a dull, brick red would result

Level 3: The typical eye color of wild type *Drosophila melanogaster*, the fruit fly, is a combination of red and brown pigments giving a dull, brick-colored red appearance.[1] While a number of different genes influence eye color in *Drosophila*, two are the focus of this question.[2] The *brown* locus (bw^+, bw) on chromosome II influences the red pigment pathway, while the *scarlet* locus (st^+, st) influences the brown pigment pathway.[3] Note: in *Drosophila*, the superscript "+" indicates wild-type alleles that are both dominant in these cases.[4] In a cross between two doubly heterozygous flies, each having dull red eyes, the following eye colors resulted in the offspring: 96 dull red, 32 brown, 29 bright red, and 11 white.[5] Provide an explanation for these results and explain why the term "novel phenotype" might apply.[6]

> Critical concepts here in that the wild-type alleles of the mutant genes will allow the red and brown pigment pathways to function

> Looks like a typical 9:3:3:1 dihybrid ratio here

Sentences 1 and 2: We imagine two pigments combining to give the dull red of wild-type, and we might diagram their synthesis and relationship below:

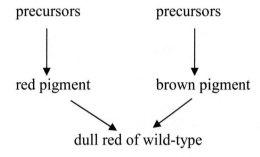

Sentence 3: This sentence sets up the critical components of the problem because it establishes the non-linked, independent relationships of the genes and the symbolism to be used.

Sentences 4 and 5: Note that the wild-type alleles allow the pathways to function to produce the red and brown pigments. We know this because the double heterozygotes each have the dull red eye color. Therefore, we have a double heterozygote ($bw^+/bw;st^+/st$) having dull red eyes. Consider the labeled pathways below:

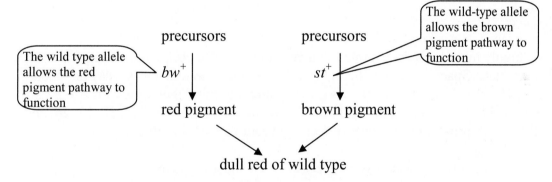

The numbers in the various phenotypes of offspring clearly follow a 9:3:3:1 ratio; therefore, the cross with genotypes of the offspring would occur in the following manner. Note: the semicolon in the symbols below is often used to symbolize that genes are on separate chromosomes.

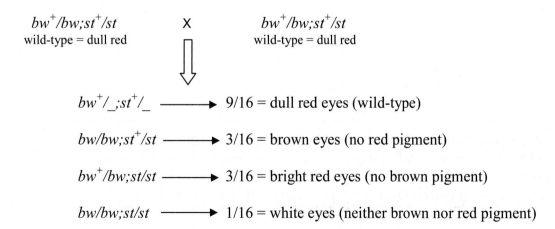

Sentence 6 and answer: The reason the description "novel phenotype" can be applied is that, unless one knew the complete chemistry of the eye color system before hand, there would be no expectation for white-eyed offspring from crosses involving dull red parents.

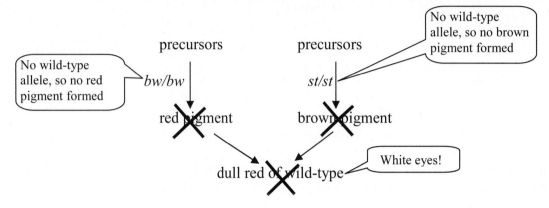

Question 11; Level 3

Theodore was a highly inbred, handsome rat with a very long tail (30 cm), while his equally inbred yet striking mate, Spacey, had a petite tail (6 cm). When Theodore and Spacey had their first litter, all had 18-cm tails. When the babies grew up and interbred, they produced 256 F2's with tails ranging in size from 6 cm to 30 cm in the following intervals: 6, 10, 14, 18, 22, 26, and 30. Of these 256 F2 offspring, four had tails of 6 cm and four had tails of 30 cm.

(a) Of the F2's, which tail length would you expect to be the most frequent?

(b) How many gene pairs appear to be influencing tail length in this example?

(c) Give the likely genotypes of Theodore and Spacey.

Concepts/Processes in Question 11: The major concept involved in this problem is **additive effects** both within and among gene pairs. The process for determining the **number of gene pairs** involved is determined by the **number of phenotypic classes** and by estimating the proportion of individuals displaying the **extreme phenotypes**.

Analysis of Question 11:

Since all the offspring had the same tail length, either the parents must have been homozygous or dominance is involved. Information in Sentences 3 and 4 will argue against dominance

"Inbred" in this context usually means homozygosity

Metric or quantitative characters often mean continuous variation

Level 3. Theodore was a highly inbred, handsome rat with a very long tail (30 cm), while his equally inbred, yet striking mate, Spacey, had a petite tail (6 cm).[1] When Theodore and Spacey had their first litter, all had 18-cm tails.[2] When the babies grew up and interbred, they produced 256 F2's with tails ranging in size from 6 cm to 30 cm in the following intervals: 6, 10, 14, 18, 22, 26, and 30.[3] Of these 256 F2 offspring, four had tails of 6 cm and four had tails of 30 cm.[4] (a) Of the F2's, which tail length would you expect to be the most frequent?[5] (b) How many gene pairs appear to be influencing tail length in this example?[6] (c) Give the likely genotypes of Theodore and Spacey.[7]

Seven classes with increments of 4

Since the extremes, 6 cm and 30 cm, have the same numbers, there must be no dominance. Four out of 256 gives 1/64 and suggests a trihybrid cross

Sentence 1: The statement that Theodore and Spacey were "highly inbred" strongly suggests that they are homozygous. Since tail length, a quantitative trait, is described, it is likely that this problem represents a case of continuous variation, where additive alleles contribute equally to the phenotype.

Sentence 2: Because the offspring all had tails of equal length (18 cm), both parents were homozygous as suggested in the first sentence. Had they been heterozygous, it is likely that varying phenotypes would have been observed in the offspring.

Sentences 3 and 4: The phenotypes of the offspring fall into seven classes, all separated by 4-cm intervals. If there are seven classes, there are likely to be three gene pairs or six alleles total, each contributing 4 cm to the phenotype. An important relationship exists between the number of classes and the number of genes, and therefore gene pairs. A general expression can be used to determine the number of genes: there will be one more class than the number of genes. So, if there are five phenotypic classes, there would be four genes, or two gene pairs. In this problem, there are seven classes, so there would be six genes, or three gene pairs. This conclusion is verified by the extreme phenotypes (6 cm and 30 cm) each having four individuals. Taking 4/256 = 1/64, which also indicates a trihybrid type of cross. Consider then that the 6-cm rats would have the *aabbcc* genotype and the 30-cm rats have the *AABBCC* genotype. Another expression that is often used to compute the number of gene pairs is $1/4^n$ = proportion of F2 individuals that express either of the extreme phenotypes. In this case, 1/64 of the rats show the extreme phenotype; therefore, there would be $n = 3$ gene pairs.

Sentence 5 and answer (a): Setting up the cross from the original to the F2 gives the following:

$$AABBCC \quad X \quad aabbcc$$
$$\text{Theodore} \quad\quad \Downarrow \quad\quad \text{Spacey}$$

$$AaBbCc \quad X \quad AaBbCc$$
$$18 \text{ cm} \quad \Downarrow \quad 18 \text{ cm}$$

In crosses involving three independently assorting gene pairs, a 64-box Punnett square could be used to describe all the gene combinations, but is not an ideal method because of the unnecessary time and labor involved. If one considers that each uppercase letter contributes a 4-cm increment to tail length (from a starting point of 6 cm), the actual distribution of phenotypes is as follows:

$$1/64 = AABBCC = \text{six uppercase letters} = 30 \text{ cm}$$
$$6/64 = \text{any combination with five uppercase letters} = 26 \text{ cm}$$
$$15/64 = \text{any combination with four uppercase letters} = 22 \text{ cm}$$
$$\mathbf{20/64 = any\ combination\ with\ three\ uppercase\ letters = 18\ cm}$$
$$15/64 = \text{any combination with two uppercase letters} = 14 \text{ cm}$$
$$6/64 = \text{any combination with one uppercase letters} = 10 \text{ cm}$$
$$1/64 = aabbcc = \text{no uppercase letters} = 6 \text{ cm}$$

The most frequent class has 18-cm tails, 20/64 or 80/256.

Sentence 6 and answer (b): (See information from Sentences 3 and 4.)

Sentence 7 and answer (c): The entire model holds together if Theodore has the genotype *AABBCC* and Spacey has the genotype *aabbcc*. Therefore, this is a case of "quantitative inheritance" with additive alleles; each upper case (but not dominant) allele contributes 4 cm of tail length.

Question 12: Level 1

Red-green colorblindness in humans is caused by a recessive gene on the X chromosome. A husband and wife both have normal vision, although both of their fathers are red-green colorblind. What is the probability that their first child will be:

(a) a son with normal vision?

(b) a daughter with normal vision?

(c) a colorblind son?

(d) a colorblind daughter?

Concepts/Processes in Question 12: This problem involves the application of **X-linked inheritance** for a recessive gene and the computation of simple probabilities.

> Females inherit an X chromosome from their father, while males inherit their X chromosome from their mother

> Females have two X chromosomes; males have an X and Y chromosome

Level 1. Red-green colorblindness in humans is caused by a recessive gene on the X chromosome.[1] A husband and wife both have normal vision, although both of their fathers are red-green colorblind.[2] What is the probability that their first child will be:[3]

    (a) a son with normal vision?
    (b) a daughter with normal vision?
    (c) a colorblind son?
    (d) a colorblind daughter?

Sentence 1: If a gene is carried on the X chromosome, females may be homozygous for the normal allele, heterozygous, or homozygous for the mutant allele. In this case, let *rg* represent the mutant allele and *Rg* represent the normal allele. Males, because they are XY, can carry only the normal allele or the mutant allele. The symbolism often used is as follows:

$$X^{Rg}X^{rg} \text{ for a heterozygous female and } X^{Rg}Y \text{ for a normal male.}$$

Sentence 2: If the husband and wife both have normal vision, they must have at least one *Rg* allele. However, since both of their fathers are colorblind, the wife must be a heterozygote because she inherits one X chromosome from her father. The husband of normal vision has the genotype $X^{Rg}Y$. The appropriate symbolism for the wife and husband is as follows:

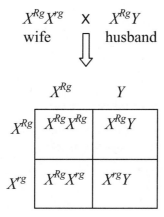

$$X^{Rg}X^{rg} \quad X \quad X^{Rg}Y$$
$$\text{wife} \quad\quad\quad \text{husband}$$

	X^{Rg}	Y
X^{Rg}	$X^{Rg}X^{Rg}$	$X^{Rg}Y$
X^{rg}	$X^{Rg}X^{rg}$	$X^{rg}Y$

Sentence 3 and answers (a)-(d): By looking at the above Punnett square, one can answer components (a)-(d) of the question.

    (a) a son with normal vision?

        The chance that the first child would be a boy with normal vision is 1/4.

    (b) a daughter with normal vision?

        The chance that the first child would be a girl with normal vision is 1/2.

    (c) a colorblind son?

        The chance that the first child would be a colorblind boy is 1/4.

    (d) a colorblind daughter?

        The chance that the first child would be a colorblind girl is zero.

Question 13: Level 4

Susan's father sufferd from Duchenne muscular dystrophy, a recessive, progressive, fatal, X-linked condition characterized by muscle wasting. Susan does not have the disease. She married John, who is also free of the disease. They have a son, Steven, with XXY (Klinefelter syndrome) and muscular dystrophy.

Describe (sketch with labeled diagrams) a single, specific chromosomal event that would account for both of Steven's afflictions (Klinefelter syndrome and muscular dystrophy).

Concepts/Processes in Question 13: This problem requires an understanding of **X-linked inheritance, meiosis,** and the consequences of **nondisjunction**.

Analysis of Question 13:

> Females have two X chromosomes: males have an X and Y chromosome

> Two "doses" are required for expression in females, and one dose in males because of the Y chromosome

Level 4. Susan's father sufferd from Duchenne muscular dystrophy, a recessive, progressive, fatal, X-linked condition characterized by muscle wasting.[1] Susan does not have the disease.[2] She married John, who is also free of the disease.[3] They have a son, Steven, with XXY (Klinefelter syndrome) and muscular dystrophy.[4] Describe (sketch with labeled diagrams) a single, specific chromosomal event that would account for both of Steven's afflictions (Klinefelter syndrome and muscular dystrophy).[5]

Sentences 1 and 2: Since Susan is free of muscular dystrophy and since females inherit one of their X chromosomes from their father, and males typically have only one X chromosome, Susan must be heterozygous: XX^{DMD} (*DMD* = gene for Duchenne muscular dystrophy).

Sentence 3: Given that the gene in question is X-linked, John must not have the *DMD* allele and therefore will be symbolized as *XY*.

Sentence 4: Steven has two X chromosomes and a Y chromosome, and he also has DMD. Clearly, nondisjunction has occurred, but in whom and at what stage? For Steven to have DMD he must have the $X^{DMD}X^{DMD}Y$ genotype and chromosomal constitution; he not only had to receive two X chromosomes from a parent, but he also must have received both *DMD* alleles.

Sentence 5: The only source of the *DMD* gene is the mother, and since Steven has two such alleles, he must have received both from the mother. Would they have come from nondisjunction at meiosis I or meiosis II? After examining the diagram below, it's clear that he must have received both <u>*DMD*</u>-containing X chromosomes from his mother, and they came from nondisjunction at meiosis II (as sister chromatids failed to separate). Steven received his Y chromosome from his father in the usual manner.

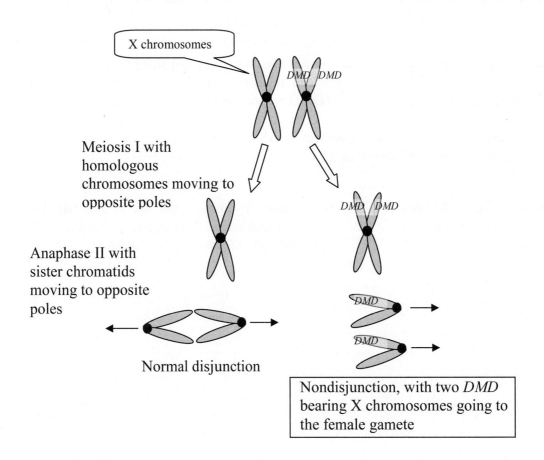

Session IV

Linkage, Crossovers, and Mapping: Where Are Genes?

Concepts/Processes	Level(s)	Relevant Question(s)	Page(s)
Linkage, two point, *cis, trans*	1	1	71
Linkage, two point, mapping	1	2	74
Mapping, data interpretation	2, 3	3, 4	76, 77
Mapping, complex symbols, probability	4	5	80
Mapping, three point, interference	3	6	82
Mapping, three point, incomplete data	4, 4	7, 8	86, 88
Reverse mapping, three point, interference	4	9	91
Pedigree with linkage, data analysis	4	10	94

Question 1: Level 1

Many loci with numerous alleles influence coat color and distribution in mammals. In rabbits, spotted (*En*) is dominant to solid (*en*), while full color or agouti (*C*) is dominant to chinchilla (c^{ch}). Rabbits that are heterozygous for both traits were crossed to solid, chinchilla rabbits and produced the following offspring:

42	solid, chinchilla
43	spotted, agouti
8	solid, agouti
7	spotted, chinchilla

(a) From the data presented above, would you consider the two loci as being *linked* or *independently assorting*?

(b) What is the arrangement of the genes in the heterozygous parent [*cis* (coupling) or *trans* (repulsion)]?

Concepts/Processes in Question 1: There are two main components to this problem. First, a **deviation from a 1:1:1:1 ratio** in the **testcross** offspring indicates **linkage**. Second, offspring data given as phenotypes and numbers indicate the *cis/trans* arrangement.

Analysis of Question 1:

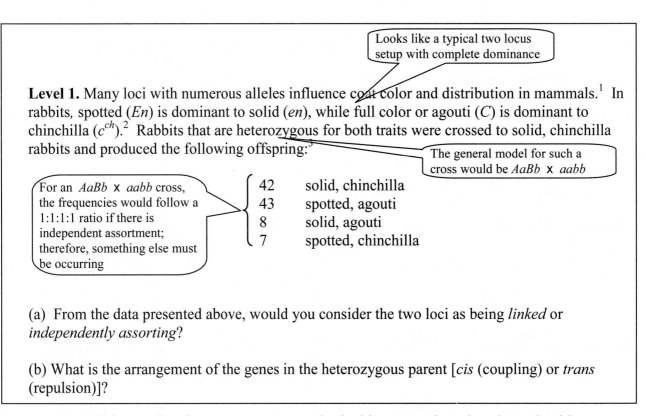

(a) From the data presented above, would you consider the two loci as being *linked* or *independently assorting*?

(b) What is the arrangement of the genes in the heterozygous parent [*cis* (coupling) or *trans* (repulsion)]?

Sentence 1: It is true that there are many coat color loci in mammals and students should expect there to be a number of interactions that include dominance, incomplete dominance, codominance, epistasis, multiple alleles, lethality, and linkage (as shown in Session III).

Sentence 2: The symbolism is standard, with dominance present at both loci. *En* is dominant to *en* and *C* is dominant to c^{ch}. Note: although not related to this question, the *C*, c^{ch} alleles are part of a string of multiple alleles at the *C* locus.

Sentence 3 and answers (a) and (b): A heterozygous spotted agouti rabbit (*En en C* c^{ch}) crossed with a solid chinchilla rabbit (*en en* c^{ch} c^{ch}) should produce offspring in a 1:1:1:1 ratio if independent assortment occurred. However, in looking at the data, clearly, the numbers do not reflect a ratio of independent assortment. The distortion could be of several origins including selective survival, sampling error, or linked genes. When examining the data, notice that the distortion from a 1:1:1:1 ratio is not random; rather, there is a pattern indicating that a reciprocal event occurred.

If one places the *En* and *C* genes on one homolog and the *en* and c^{ch} genes on the other, the two most frequent classes in the offspring can be accounted for as indicated below:

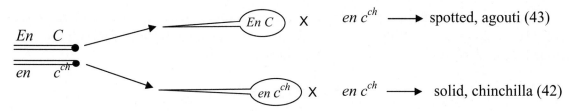

In this case the "parental" arrangement has been maintained when gametes are formed.

But what about the other two classes of offspring? If you place a crossover between the two loci as shown below, the other two classes can be accounted for.

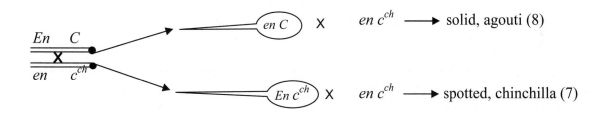

Therefore, the most likely explanation for the numbers given in the offspring is that the two loci are linked (on the same homolog) and some crossing over occurred to break up the linkage arrangement. In other words, **exceptional** or **recombinant** gametes have been produced as a result of crossing over and the results are reciprocal in that for every exceptional gamete of the solid, agouti type (8 of them), there is a similar number of the spotted, chinchilla type (7).

Notice that in the illustrations presented above, the dominant alleles are on one homolog while the recessive alleles are on the other. When this arrangement occurs, it is called "*cis*" or "*coupling*." This is an important concept to master and will be dealt with again in Question 2. After working through Question 2, you will see the importance of understanding the concepts of "*cis*" and "*trans*" when dealing with linkage problems.

As in the above question, in rabbits, spotted (*En*) is dominant to solid (*en*), while full color or agouti (*C*) is dominant to chinchilla (*c^ch*). Rabbits that are heterozygous for both traits were crossed to solid, chinchilla rabbits with the following results:

> 8 solid, chinchilla
> 6 spotted, agouti
> 45 solid, agouti
> 41 spotted, chinchilla

(a) What is the arrangement of the genes in the heterozygous parent [*cis* (coupling) or *trans* (repulsion)]?

(b) What is the map distance between the two loci?

Concepts/Processes in Question 2: The main components in this problem involve a determination of the *cis/trans* arrangement in the heterozygous parent and an understanding of **chromosome mapping**.

Analysis of Question 2:

Level 1. As in the above question, in rabbits, spotted (*En*) is dominant to solid (*en*), while full color or agouti (*C*) is dominant to chinchilla (*c^ch*).[1] Rabbits that are heterozygous for both traits were crossed to solid, chinchilla rabbits with the following results:[2]

> 8 solid, chinchilla
> 6 spotted, agouti
> 45 solid, agouti
> 41 spotted, chinchilla

Take a quick glance at the results from the cross in Question 1 above. Note the difference

(a) What is the arrangement of the genes in the heterozygous parent [*cis* (coupling) or *trans* (repulsion)] ?

(b) What is the map distance between the two loci?

Sentence 1: (Same as Sentence 2 in Question 1) It is true that there are many coat color loci in mammals, and students should expect there to be a number of interactions including dominance, incomplete dominance, codominance, epistasis, multiple alleles, lethality, and linkage (as shown in Session III). The symbolism is standard, with dominance present at both loci. *En* is dominant to *en* and *C* is dominant to c^{ch}.

Sentence 2 and answers (a) and (b): Notice that the distribution of offspring is reversed from that in Question 1. This is extremely important when dealing with linkage issues because it is the position of genes on chromosomes that is sought and that can't be determined accurately without knowledge of the arrangement of those genes. Notice the difference between the diagram below and the diagram in Question 1 above.

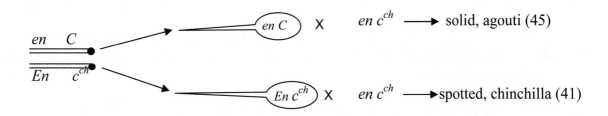

Accounting for all the phenotypic classes, below is a figure indicating the recombinant or exceptional gametes through crossing over.

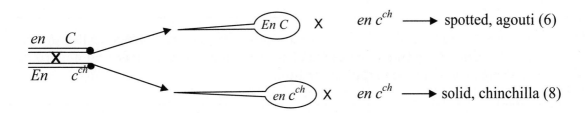

So, for answer (a), fully accounting for the phenotypes and their frequencies places the original parental arrangement in the *trans* or *repulsion* arrangement, where each homolog has a recessive and a dominant gene. Again, this may seem like a trivial issue, but it is not --- the meaning of "*cis*" and "*trans*" is very important in mapping genes (see below) because it allows one to identify noncrossover offspring (so-called parentals) and the recombinant offspring.

Determining the map distance between the two loci (answer b) is straightforward if one can identify the noncrossover and recombinant offspring. Study the following simple expression.

Map distance (recombination frequency) =

Number of recombinant offspring   X 100 (to convert to a percentage)
        Total number of offspring

In this question, there are 14 recombinant offspring (crossover between the two loci) and 100 total offspring.

$$\text{Map distance} = \frac{14}{100} \times 100 = 14.0$$

Mapping the *En* and *C* loci in this problem was straightforward. Stay tuned: there are complications coming.

Question 3: Level 2

Assume that a cross is made between *AaBb* and *aabb* plants and the offspring occur in the following numbers: 106 *AaBb*, 48 *Aabb*, 52 *aaBb*, and 94 *aabb*. These results are consistent with which following circumstance?

    A.   X-linked inheritance with 30% crossing over
    B.   linkage with 50% crossing over
    C.   linkage with approximately 33 map units between the two gene loci
    D.   independent assortment
    E.   linked with 100 map units between the two gene loci

Concepts/Processes in Question 3: To solve this problem, one must recognize that the data do not fit a **1:1:1:1** ratio. **Mapping** requires the identification of the **crossover and noncrossover** offspring and application of the **mapping formula**.

Analysis of Question 3:

Level 2. Assume that a cross is made between *AaBb* and *aabb* plants and the offspring occur in the following numbers: 106 *AaBb*, 48 *Aabb*, 52 *aaBb*, and 94 *aabb*.[1] These results are consistent with which following circumstance?[2]

                      Data indicate a significant departure from a 1:1:1:1 ratio

    A.   X-linked inheritance with 30% crossing over
    B.   linkage with 50% crossing over
    C.   linkage with approximately 33 map units between the two gene loci
    D.   independent assortment
    E.   linked with 100 map units between the two gene loci

Sentence 1: This is a typical backcross (or testcross) setup with a double heterozygote crossed to a fully recessive plant. If independent assortment occurred, then there would be approximately equal numbers in each class of offspring. However, in looking at the data, clearly, a 1:1:1:1 ratio does not exist (which a chi-Square analysis would demonstrate). Therefore, something other than independent assortment is operating, and there is no indication of an X-linked relationship in either the initial setup or the data. If either gene occupied the X chromosome, there would not be two alleles present at each locus.

Sentence 2 and answer: We are looking for linkage (absence of independent assortment) and no X-linkage, so choices A and D are eliminated. Choice B is interesting in that it is internally conflicted. If you have linkage, there must be less than 50% crossing over, because with 50% crossing over, you have independent assortment. Think about it: if half of the offspring are recombinant and half are parental, you have a 1:1:1:1 ratio, which is independent assortment.

Now for choice E: the number 100 comes from the sum of the two recombinant classes. To map genes, one must divide by the total number of offspring, which in this case is 300. Therefore, choice E is not viable. We are left with choice C in which there are 33 map units between the two loci. Applying the formula described for mapping in Question 2 above:

$$\frac{\text{Number of recombinant offspring}}{\text{Total number of offspring}} \quad X \ 100 \ (\text{to convert to a percentage})$$

$$\frac{48 + 52}{300} \quad X \ 100 \ = \ \text{about 33\% or 33 map units}$$

The correct answer is therefore **C**.

Question 4: Level 3

The genes for *mahogany eyes* and *ebony body* are approximately 25 map units apart on chromosome III in *Drosophila*. Assume that a mahogany-eyed female was mated to an ebony-bodied male and the resulting F1 phenotypically wild-type females were mated to mahogany, ebony males. Of 1000 offspring, what would be the expected phenotypes and in what numbers would they be expected?

Phenotypes	**Expected Number**
_____	_____
_____	_____
_____	_____
_____	_____

Concepts/Processes in Question 4: This problem requires a mastery of the concept of **linkage** as determined from **testcross data**. It also requires an understanding of **map units** and the manner in which map units are obtained. An understanding of *cis/trans* arrangements is required and how such arrangements affect the outcome of crosses involving linkage.

Analysis of Question 4:

We have a cross between two mutant strains; that immediately sets up an F1 in *trans*. In addition, both mutant genes are recessive (because the F1s are wild-type) and all the parents are homozygous

We know that this is a linkage problem because the map units are given (and are less than 50). Genes are not X-linked

Level 3. The genes for *mahogany eyes* and *ebony body* are approximately 25 map units apart on chromosome III in *Drosophila*.[1] Assume that a mahogany-eyed female was mated to an ebony-bodied male and the resulting F1 phenotypically wild-type females were mated to mahogany, ebony males.[2] Of 1000 offspring, what would be the expected phenotypes and in what numbers would they be expected?[3]

Phenotypes	Expected Number
_____	_____
_____	_____
_____	_____
_____	_____

This question is the reverse of previous questions. In this case, you are given the map units and total number of offspring and you must come up with the expected numbers that gave the 25 map units

Sentence 1: Here the map units are given, and since chromosome III is involved, the genes are not X-linked.

Sentence 2: If a mutant female (mahogany eyes) is mated to a mutant male (ebony body) and all the offspring are wild-type, we know that the mahogany and ebony genes are recessive and that both parents are homozygous. We also know that the gene arrangement is *trans* because each mutant gene is coming in from a different parent. See the diagram below for an explanation. Notice that the F1 females were mated to the doubly homozygous males. Given that crossing over in *Drosophila* only occurs in females, significantly different results would have occurred if the reciprocal cross were conducted. In other words, since there is no crossing over in male *Drosophila*, the two genes would show complete linkage if the reciprocal cross occurred (heterozygous male crossed with double mutant female).

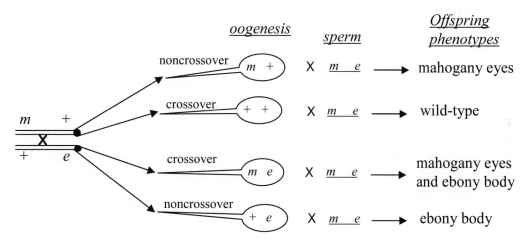

Sentence 3 and answer: Examine the above figure and notice that there are two "parental" (nonrecombinant) classes: mahogany eyes at the top and ebony body at the bottom. Also notice that there are two recombinant classes: the center two of the four listed (wild-type and mahogany/ebony). Since the map distance between the two loci is 25 map units, the recombinant classes must add up to 25% of the total. The total number of offspring is 1000. So, there must have been 250 recombinant offspring, 125 each of the two recombinant classes. If that's the case, there would be a total of 750 nonrecombinants: 375 in each of the two classes. So the answers for the table would be as follows:

Phenotypes	Expected Number	
mahogany eyes	375	
wild-type	125	⎱ recombinant classes
mahogany/ebony	125	⎰
ebony body	375	

One of the most common mistakes that students make with this type of problem is not seeing that the F1 female gene arrangement is in *trans* rather than *cis*. On your own, consider a rewording of the problem that would put the F1 female gene arrangement in *cis*. This is a very important concept for you to master.

The *Xg* locus on the human X chromosome has two alleles, a^+ and a. The a^+ allele causes the presence of the Xg surface protein on red blood cells, while the recessive a allele does not allow the antigen to appear. The *Xg* locus is about 10 map units (centimorgans) from the *STS* locus. The *STS* locus produces normal steroid sulfatase activity, while its recessive *sts* allele results in lack of steroid sulfatase activity. Individuals with one form of scaly skin (X-linked ichthyosis) have the *sts/sts* genotype (*sts*/Y if male). A man with ichthyosis and no *Xg* antigen has a normal daughter with Xg antigen, who is expecting a child.

(a) If the child is a boy, what is the probability that he will lack the Xg antigen and have ichthyosis?

(b) What is the probability that a son would have both the antigen and ichthyosis?

Concepts/Processes in Question 5: There are several main concepts in this question. One must master **complex symbolism**, understand the origin of a *cis* or *trans* gene arrangement, and incorporate **map units** in the solution.

Analysis of Question 5:

> To this point, it appears as a dihybrid arrangement because two loci have been described, both on the X chromosome and 10 unites apart

Level 4. The *Xg* locus on the human X chromosome has two alleles, a^+ and a.[1] The a^+ allele causes the presence of the Xg surface protein on red blood cells, while the recessive a allele does not allow the antigen to appear.[2] The *Xg* locus is about 10 map units (centimorgans) from the *STS* locus.[3] The *STS* locus produces normal steroid sulfatase activity, while its recessive *sts* allele results in lack of steroid sulfatase activity.[4] Individuals with one form of scaly skin (X-linked ichthyosis) have the *sts/sts* genotype (*sts*/Y if male).[5] A man with ichthyosis and no *Xg* antigen has a normal daughter with Xg antigen, who is expecting a child.[6]

> This sentence is the meat of the question

> Interesting point but really not important in terms of solving the problem

(a) If the child is a boy, what is the probability that he will lack the Xg antigen and have ichthyosis?

(b) What is the probability that a son would have both the antigen and ichthyosis?

Note: This is a wordy question by design. The best way to approach such a problem is to apply what you know and focus on fundamentals.

Sentences 1 and 2: There are two alleles, a^+ and a, at the *Xg* locus, simple as that. If an individual has the $a+$ allele, he or she has the Xg antigen on the red blood cell surface. Because the locus is X-linked, females can be a^+/a^+, a^+/a, or a/a. Males can be either a^+/Y or a/Y.

Sentence 3: The *STS* locus, being 10 map units away, sets up a linkage problem in that crossing over is going to recombine the genes at the two loci and give rise to four different arrangements in the gametes. The solution to this problem, once set up correctly, is no different from earlier problems in this section. There are no new concepts that come into play --- its solution is based solely on the application of proper symbolism and linkage with two X-linked genes.

Sentences 4 and 5: Sentence 4, while interesting, adds nothing to the solution of the problem. It merely describes some of the cell biology associated with this form of ichthyosis. Sentence 5 tells us that the *sts* allele is recessive because it only describes the *sts/sts* genotype as being associated with the skin condition.

Sentence 6: This is the critical setup portion of the question. A man with ichthyosis (must be *sts/Y*) and no Xg antigen (must be *a/Y*) has a normal daughter with Xg antigen. Because there are 10 map units between the two loci, each of the two crossover classes would constitute 5%. The daughter must have the following genetic arrangement on her X chromosomes:

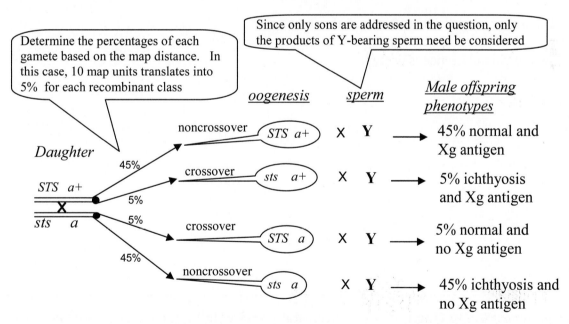

Answer to part (a): From the figure above, the probability that "he will lack the Xg antigen and have ichthyosis" is 45%. Answer to part (b): Again, from the figure above, the "probability that a son would have both the antigen and ichthyosis" is 5%.

In most cases, students are unsure of what to do with the 10 map units between the two genes.

In *Drosophila*, a fully heterozygous female with the X-linked recessive genes *a*, *b*, and *c* (not necessarily in that order on the chromosome) was mated to a male that was genetically *a, b, c* (not necessarily in that order on the chromosome). The offspring occurred in the following phenotypic ratios:

Phenotypes	Numbers
wild	426
a,c,b	428
a	23
c,b	22
c	49
b, a	46
b	3
c, a	2
Total	1000

(a) What is the *cis/trans* arrangement among the genes?

(b) Regarding the arrangement of genes on the chromosome, which gene is in the middle?

(c) What are the map distances between the three loci?

(d) How much interference is present?

Concepts/Processes in Question 6: To successfully answer this question, one must understand *cis/trans* arrangements and how to determine which **gene is in the middle** from actual data. One must be able to compute a **coefficient of coincidence** and **interference**.

Analysis of Question 6

Level 3. In *Drosophila*, a fully heterozygous female with the X-linked recessive genes *a*, *b*, and *c* (not necessarily in that order on the chromosome) was mated to a male that was genetically *a, b, c* (not necessarily in that order on the chromosome).[1] The offspring occurred in the following phenotypic ratios:[2]

> At this point, we don't know the *cis/trans* arrangements of these genes

> This is a typical trihybrid backcross or testcross

Phenotypes	Numbers
wild	426
a,c,b	428
a	23
c,b	22
c	49
b, a	46
b	3
c, a	2
Total	1000

(a) What is the *cis/trans* arrangement among the genes?

(b) Regarding the arrangement of genes on the chromosome, which gene is in the middle?

(c) What are the map distances between the three loci?

(d) How much interference is present?

Sentence 1: At this point in the description, there is no indication of the gene order or the *cis/trans* arrangements. Both are critical in answering parts (a), (b), (c), and (d). The data will provide both necessary components.

Sentence 2: There are three basic procedures to follow when getting started. First, be certain that there are eight classes represented in the offspring. Because this is a trihybrid cross, there should be eight classes. This will sound strange, but if there are less than eight (six, for example; see below), determine which ones are missing, add them to the list, and then enter zeros for their numbers. You will see why this is necessary in subsequent questions.

Now, for part (a), determine the *cis/trans* arrangement of the genes. Notice that the wild-type and the triple mutant phenotypes are the most frequent. These are the noncrossover (or parental) offspring. If the genes were in the *cis* arrangement as indicated below, one would expect the wild and triple mutant phenotypes to be the most frequent. Since that is what is observed, the genes must all be in the *cis* arrangement.

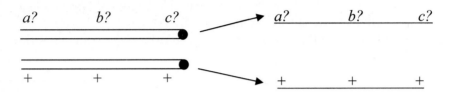

For part (b), we must decide which gene is in the middle. The best way to determine gene order is to look at the double crossover classes (least frequent) and compare them to the parental (noncrossover) classes. Ask yourself which gene switched places. The gene that switches places when comparing the parental with the double crossover classes will be the gene in the middle. Notice that gene b switches places. Therefore, it must be in the middle. Once the gene arrangement has been determined, rewrite the sequence and identify the two crossover regions as region I and region II, as shown below:

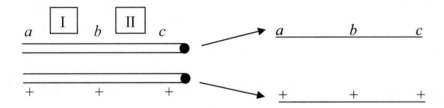

For part (c), consider that the map distance is a summation of the crossover frequency between two loci. So determining the map distance between *a* and *b,* would be as follows:

Region I: Map units between *a* and *b* = $\dfrac{23 + 22 + 3 + 2}{1000}$ X 100 = $\dfrac{50}{1000}$ = 5

At this point, you might be wondering about the addition of 3 + 2 in the above equation. Remember, map units attempt to assess the crossover frequency between two points. Since each double crossover involved a crossover in region I, they must be added to the mapping function.

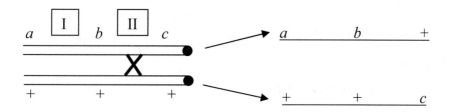

Region II: Map units between b and c = $\dfrac{49 + 46 + 3 + 2}{1000}$ X 100   = $\dfrac{100}{1000}$ = 10

So the map, its arrangement and distances are now complete.

For part (d), we need to determine the coefficient of coincidence, from which we will determine the interference. Interference is 1.0 minus the coefficient of coincidence.

The coefficient of coincidence is determined by relating the frequency of double crossovers observed to the frequency expected. The observed number of double crossovers is 5; therefore, the frequency is 5/1000 or 0.005. The expected frequency of double crossovers is 0.05 (frequency of crossovers in region I) X 0.10 (frequency of crossovers in region II) = 0.005. So, the coefficient of coincidence is as follows:

Coefficient of coincidence = $\dfrac{(5/1000)}{0.05 \text{ X } 0.10}$ = $\dfrac{0.005}{0.005}$ = 1.0

The interference, 1.0 minus the coefficient of coincidence, therefore is zero. This means that there were as many double crossovers as expected. One crossover did not interfere with neighboring crossovers.

In *Drosophila*, a fully heterozygous female with the X-linked recessive traits *a*, *b*, and *c* (not necessarily in that order on the chromosome) was mated to a male that was genetically *a*, *b*, and *c* (not necessarily in that order on the chromosome). The following phenotypes with their respective numbers resulted from the mating:

Phenotypes			Numbers
+	b	+	12
+	+	c	680
a	+	c	14
a	b	+	667
a	+	+	16
+	b	c	12
		Total	1401

(a) Regarding the arrangement of genes on the chromosome, which gene is in the middle and what is the *cis/trans* arrangement?

(b) How much interference occurred?

Concepts/Processes in Question 7: This problem requires a determination of **gene order** where there are **no double crossover progeny** listed. In addition, a **shortcut** is available for those knowing how the **coefficient of coincidence** is calculated. The **interference** value is easily determined without calculations

Analysis of Question 7:

Level 4 In *Drosophila*, a fully heterozygous female with the X-linked recessive traits *a*, *b*, and *c* (not necessarily in that order on the chromosome) was mated to a male that was genetically *a*, *b*, and *c* (not necessarily in that order on the chromosome).[1] The following phenotypes with their respective numbers resulted from the mating:[2]

> Introduction identical to that of Question 6 above

Phenotypes			Numbers
+	b	+	12
+	+	c	680
a	+	c	14
a	b	+	667
a	+	+	16
+	b	c	12
		Total	1401

> Notice that all the eight classes are not listed. There are two classes missing

(a) Regarding the arrangement of genes on the chromosome, which gene is in the middle and what is the *cis/trans* arrangement? (b) How much interference occurred?

Sentence 1: At this point in the description, there is no indication of the gene order or the *cis/trans* arrangements. Notice that this time, the map distances are not being requested, as they are in Question 6 above.

Sentence 2: As stated in Question 6 above, there are three basic procedures to follow when getting started with these types of questions. First, be certain that there are eight classes represented in the offspring. Notice that there are only six listed. Because this is a trihybrid cross, there should be eight classes. Sometimes, if the loci are close together and the sample size is relatively small, double crossover individuals are not represented. Determine which classes are missing, then add them to the list and place zeros for their numbers.

Phenotypes			Numbers
+	b	+	12
+	+	c	680
a	+	c	14
a	b	+	667
a	+	+	16
+	b	c	12
a	b	c	0
+	+	+	0
		Total	1401

> These values were added to complete the data set and facilitate determining gene order and the *cis/trans* relationships

For part (a), we must decide which gene is in the middle. The best way to determine gene order is to look at the double crossover classes (least frequent --- zeros in this case) and compare them to the parental (noncrossover) classes. Ask yourself which gene switched places. The gene that switches places when comparing the parental with the double crossover classes will be the gene in the middle. Notice that gene *c* switches places. Therefore, it (gene *c*) must be in the middle. Once the gene arrangement has been determined, rewrite the sequence.

Now that the gene sequence is determined, the *cis/trans* arrangement can be addressed. Notice that the parentals (noncrossovers = the most abundant) are *++c* and *ab+*. Because the noncrossover classes represent the parental arrangement (that's why they are called "parentals"), we can easily see the *cis/trans* arrangement, as indicated below:

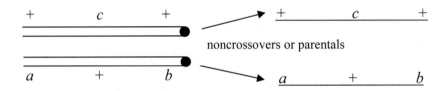

Part (a) of the question is answered: gene *c* is in the middle and *a-c* are in *trans*, *c-b* are in *trans*, and *a-b* are in *cis*.

For part (b), consider that there are no double crossovers; we added them as zeros to complete the data set. If there are no double crossovers, the coefficient of coincidence is zero. If the coefficient of coincidence is zero, the interference is 1.0, which makes sense because no double crossovers were observed (i.e., 100% interference).

Question 8: Level 4

A cross is made between a triply heterozygous female and a triply homozygous mutant male *Drosophila* containing the genes (not necessarily in this order) *prune*, *vermilion*, and *brown*. Offspring occurred in the following frequencies:

purple, brown (46)   purple (347)   purple, vermilion (97)
brown (103)   vermilion (54)   vermilion, brown (353)

(a) Which gene is in the middle?

(b) What is the *purple-vermilion* map distance?

(c) What is the interference value?

Concepts/Processes in Question 8: While this is a **trihybrid cross**, there are several **complexities**. First, **phenotypes are provided**, thereby requiring the development of **appropriate symbols**. Second, there are **no double crossover progeny** in the data set, thereby indicating **complete interference**. The parental female has a mix of *cis* and *trans* gene arrangements.

Analysis of Question 8:

Actual data being presented, but still a typical trihybrid backcross

Level 4. A cross is made between a triply heterozygous female and a triply homozygous mutant male *Drosophila* containing the genes (not necessarily in this order): *prune, vermilion,* and *brown.*[1] Offspring occurred in the following frequencies:[2]

purple, brown (46)	purple (347)	purple, vermilion (97)
brown (103)	vermilion (54)	vermilion, brown (353)

(a) Which gene is in the middle?

A different format is given but it will still be addressed as in the more generic Question #6 above

(b) What is the *purple-vermilion* map distance?

(c) What is the interference value?

Sentence 1: Notice that the setup for this problem is the same as in Question 6 above; however, the data are presented in a different format and actual mutants are used. You should approach the problem the same way as Question 6 above.

Sentence 2: Notice that only six classes are presented. In general, the double crossover classes are missing --- they are the least frequent and may be zero if the map distances are short and/or there is considerable interference. Therefore, determine the classes missing and add them (with zeros).*

purple, brown (46)	purple (347)	purple, vermilion (97)
brown (103)	vermilion (54)	vermilion, brown (353)
*wild (0)	*purple, vermilion, brown (0)	

Compare the double crossover classes (wild and purple, vermilion, brown in this case) to the parental classes (the most frequent = purple and vermilion, brown) and determine which gene switched places. In this case (a), the *purple* gene switched and is therefore in the middle. Rewrite the sequence as indicated below; however, to answer part (b) the *cis/trans* arrangement must be determined. Examine the parental classes and couple that information with your conclusion that the *purple* gene is in the middle.

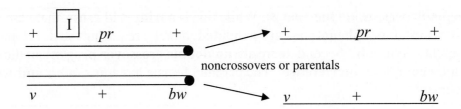

For determining the *purple-vermilion* map distance, region I above, consider the following products:

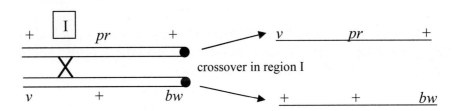

So, we should look for classes purple-vermilion and brown. Looking at the data above we see classes purple-vermilion (97) and brown (103). In general, unless there is some sort of epistasis occurring, the numbers should be similar, as 97 and 103 are in this case. Mapping can proceed as follows:

> For consistency, include the zero values even though they do not affect the map distance

Region I: Map units between *pr* and *v* = $\dfrac{97 + 103 + 0 + 0}{1000}$ X 100 = $\dfrac{200}{1000}$ = 20

Therefore, the answer for part (b) is 20 map units.

For part (c), consider that there are no double crossovers; we added them as zeros to complete the data set. If there are no double crossovers, the coefficient of coincidence is zero. If the coefficient of coincidence is zero, interference is 1.0, which makes sense because no double crossovers were observed (i.e., 100% interference).

Question 9: Level 4

The following represents the approximate map positions of three genes found on human chromosome 9:

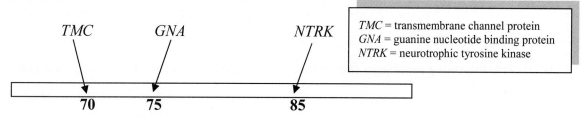

TMC   GNA   NTRK

TMC = transmembrane channel protein
GNA = guanine nucleotide binding protein
NTRK = neurotrophic tyrosine kinase

70   75   85

Assume that a female is *cis* heterozygous for all three of these loci. She produces 4000 gametes. Given a coefficient of coincidence of 0.50, what gametes would she be expected to produce and how many of each type? Please list them below under the appropriate headings.

Gamete genotype   *Number expected*

Concepts/Processes in Question 9: This problem provides the **map distances** among the three loci and asks for **gametic frequencies** that produced those map distances. This is the **reverse** of often-used **three point mapping** problems. A **coefficient of coincidence** is given, from which one can calculate the **expected numbers** of **double crossover** gametes. Other **crossover and parental gametes** are then calculated. An appropriate **symbol set** is expected.

Analysis of Question 9:

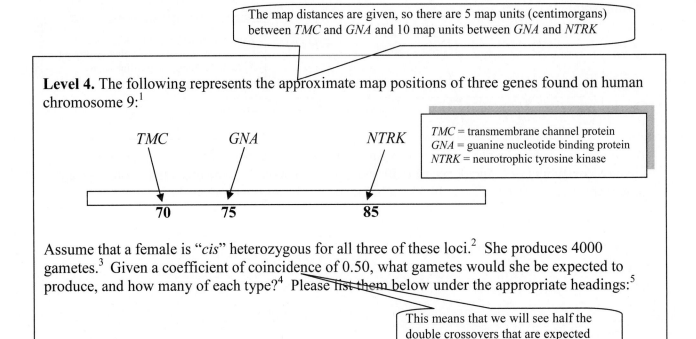

The map distances are given, so there are 5 map units (centimorgans) between *TMC* and *GNA* and 10 map units between *GNA* and *NTRK*

Level 4. The following represents the approximate map positions of three genes found on human chromosome 9:[1]

TMC   GNA   NTRK

TMC = transmembrane channel protein
GNA = guanine nucleotide binding protein
NTRK = neurotrophic tyrosine kinase

70   75   85

Assume that a female is "*cis*" heterozygous for all three of these loci.[2] She produces 4000 gametes.[3] Given a coefficient of coincidence of 0.50, what gametes would she be expected to produce, and how many of each type?[4] Please list them below under the appropriate headings:[5]

This means that we will see half the double crossovers that are expected

Gamete genotype   *Number expected*

Sentence 1: The gene sequence and map distances are given; the question will ask for the number of organisms in each class that would give these map distances.

Sentences 2 and 3: All the genes are in the *cis* arrangement, and 4000 gametes are produced; therefore, we can merely work backwards (from a typical mapping problem) to determine how many are expected in each class. Start with the double crossover class.

Sentence 4 and 5, and answer: If the coefficient of coincidence is 0.5, the following expression will allow us to determine the observed number:

$$\text{Coefficient of coincidence} = \frac{\text{observed double crossovers}}{\text{expected double crossovers}}$$

$$0.5 = \frac{\text{observed double crossovers}}{0.05 \ \times \ 0.10 \ \times \ 4000}$$

> These values come from the map units between the gene pairs. Because there are 5 map units between *TMC* and *GNA*, the probability of a crossover is 0.05. The same logic is applied for the second interval to arrive at 0.10

$$0.5 = \frac{\text{observed double crossovers}}{20}$$

$$\text{observed double crossovers} = 0.5 \ \times \ 20 \ = \ 10$$

So, there are 10 double crossovers, but since there are two kinds of double crossover classes, there would be 5 in each, as shown in the table below:

Event	*Gamete genotype*	*Number expected*
Noncrossover	TMC GNA NTRK	1705
	tmc gna ntrk	1705
Crossover in region I	*TMC gna ntrk*	95
	tmc GNA NTRK	95
Crossover in region II	*TMC GNA ntrk*	195
	tmc gna NTRK	195
Crossover in regions I and II	*TMC gna NTRK*	5
	tmc GNA ntrk	5

For the gametes with crossovers in region I, there are 5 map units, so 0.05 x 4000 = 200, but one must subtract the double crossovers (because they were added when arriving at the 5 map units). Therefore, 200 - 10 = 190, and dividing by 2 for the two types within the region I crossover class gives 95 each.

For the gametes with crossovers in region II, there are 10 map units, so 0.10 x 4000 = 400, but one must subtract the double crossovers (because they were added with arriving at the 10 map units). Therefore, 400 - 10 = 390, and dividing by 2 for the two types within the region II crossover class gives 195 each.

To determine the numbers in the parental class, add all the region I, region II, and double crossover numbers together and subtract that number from the total. Dividing by 2 gives each of the noncrossover gametes (4000 – 590 = 3410, dividing by 2 gives 1705 each).

When completing such a problem, add all the components to see if they sum to the total number of gametes or offspring.

Question 10: Level 4

The *Xg* locus on the human X chromosome has two alleles, a^+ and *a*. The a^+ allele causes the presence of the Xg surface protein on red blood cells, while the recessive *a* allele does not allow the antigen to appear. The *Xg* locus is about 10 map units (centimorgans) from the *STS* locus. Individuals with one form of scaly skin (X-linked ichthyosis) have the *sts/sts* genotype (*sts*/Y if male). A man with ichthyosis and no Xg antigen has a normal daughter with Xg antigen who marries a normal man with no Xg antigen. They have five children of the following phenotypes:

Female	=	normal, Xg antigen present
Male	=	normal, Xg antigen present
Male	=	ichthyosis, no Xg antigen
Female	=	normal, no Xg antigen
Male	=	normal, no Xg antigen

(a) Construct a pedigree that reflects the relationships and phenotypes described above.

(b) Of the five children listed above, state who have phenotypes resulting from a crossover, who have phenotypes that did not involve a crossover, and for whom it would be impossible to determine whether or not a crossover occurred.

Concepts/Processes in Question 10: There are several major issues to deal with in this problem. First, arriving at an appropriate *cis* **symbolism** is necessary for setting up the solution. Second, one must see that the stated **map units (10) are not required** for the solution of this problem. Third, a **pedigree** is required that symbolizes the statements in the question and allows one to more easily work out its solution. An understanding of **X-linked inheritance** is necessary.

Analysis of Question 10:

Level 4. The *Xg* locus on the human X chromosome has two alleles, a^+ and a.[1] The a^+ allele causes the presence of the Xg surface protein on red blood cells, while the recessive a allele does not allow the antigen to appear.[2] The *Xg* locus is about 10 map units (centimorgans) from the *STS* locus.[3] Individuals with one form of scaly skin (X-linked ichthyosis) have the *sts/sts* genotype (*sts*/Y if male).[4] A man with ichthyosis and no Xg antigen has a normal daughter with Xg antigen who marries a normal man with no Xg antigen.[5] They have five children of the following phenotypes:[6]

Female	=	normal, Xg antigen present
Male	=	normal, Xg anitgen present
Male	=	ichthyosis, no Xg antigen
Female	=	normal, no Xg antigen
Male	=	normal, no Xg antigen

Since this is a fairly wordy description of the problem, it would be best to lay out the genotypes in these individuals in the form of a pedigree

(a) Construct a pedigree that reflects the relationships and phenotypes described above.

(b) Of the five children listed above, state who have phenotypes resulting from a crossover, who have phenotypes that did not involve a crossover, and for whom it would be impossible to determine whether or not a crossover occurred.

Sentences 1 and 2: There are two alleles, a^+ and *a,* at the *Xg* locus, simple as that. If an individual has the a^+ allele, he or she has the Xg antigen on the red blood cell surface. Because the locus is X-linked, females can be a^+/a^+, a^+/a, or *a/a*. Males can be either a^+/Y or *a*/Y.

Sentence 3 and 4: The *STS* locus, being 10 map units away, sets up a linkage problem in that crossing over is going to recombine the genes at the two loci and give rise to four different arrangements in the gametes. The solution to this problem, once set up correctly, is no different from that of earlier problems in this section. There are no new concepts that come into play --- its solution is based solely on the application of proper symbolism and linkage with two X-linked genes.

Sentence 5 and 6, and answer (a): This is the critical part of the problem. We will set up the pedigree but also add the chromosomal/genetic setup so that correct answers are clearly visible.

The man with ichthyosis and no Xg antigen would contribute the following X chromosome to his daughter: <u>*sts   a*</u>

The man's normal daughter must have the following genotype: <u>*STS   a⁺*</u>
$\qquad\qquad\qquad\qquad\qquad\qquad\qquad\qquad\qquad\qquad\qquad$ *sts   a*

> This is the chromosome that the daughter inherited from her father, the other chromosome must have been a *cis STS a⁺*.

The normal daughter (above) marries a normal man with no Xg antigen, so her husband has the following genotype: <u>*STS a*</u>
$\qquad\qquad\qquad\qquad\qquad\qquad\qquad\qquad\quad$ Y

The marriage that produced the five children appears as follows:

$$\frac{\underline{STS\ \ a^+}}{sts\ \ \ a} \quad \times \quad \frac{\underline{STS\ \ a}}{Y}$$

For answer (a), the pedigree is as follows:

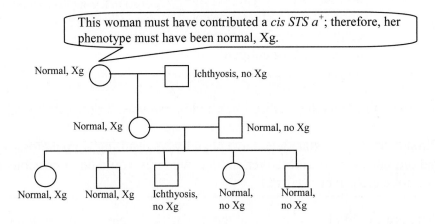

> This woman must have contributed a *cis STS a⁺*; therefore, her phenotype must have been normal, Xg.

By considering the genetic alignment in chromosome 9 for individuals that produced the five children, one can see how the answers (below) were determined.

$$\frac{\underline{STS\ \ a^+}}{sts\ \ \ a} \quad \times \quad \frac{\underline{STS\ \ a}}{Y}$$

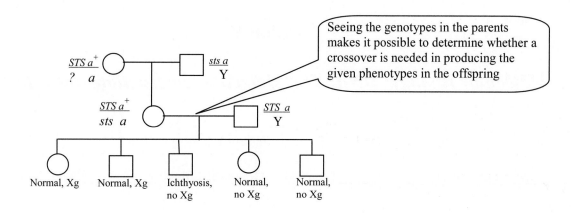

Seeing the genotypes in the parents makes it possible to determine whether a crossover is needed in producing the given phenotypes in the offspring

Normal, Xg Normal, Xg Ichthyosis, no Xg Normal, no Xg Normal, no Xg

Answers

Female	=	normal, Xg antigen present	impossible to determine
Male	=	normal, Xg anitgen present	no crossover need occur
Male	=	ichthyosis, no Xg antigen	no crossover need occur
Female	=	normal, no Xg antigen	impossible to determine
Male	=	normal, no Xg antigen	crossing over occurred

Session V

Molecular Biology: DNA: The Molecular Instructions for Life

Two lines of direct evidence and two lines of indirect evidence indicated that DNA is the genetic material in prokaryotes and eukaryotes and many viruses. A line of work beginning with Griffith (1927) and ending with Avery, MacLeod, and McCarty (1944) supported the hypothesis that DNA is the genetic material in *Pneumococci,* while Hershey and Chase (1952) provided supporting results with phage T2. Indirect evidence came from comparisons of DNA content in haploid and diploid cells and the mutagenesis spectrum generated by exposure to ultraviolet light.

(a) Griffith discovered that *Streptococcus pneumonia* (*Pneumococci*) caused pneumonia in mice. In his experiments, mice were injected with different strains of treated and untreated bacteria. For each of the following, indicate whether the mice *lived* or *died*.

$$\textit{\textbf{lived or died?}}$$

   (1) mice injected with living III*S* (virulent)   _____
   (2) mice injected with living II*R* (avirulent)   _____
   (3) mice injected with heat-killed II*R*   _____
   (4) mice injected with heat-killed III*S*   _____
   (5) mice injected with living II*R* + heat-killed III*S*   _____
   (6) mice injected with living III*S* + heat-killed II*R*   _____

(b) When Avery *et al.* developed an extract from III*S* (virulent) cells and removed proteins by several chloroform extractions, transformation of II*R* (*occurred* or *failed to occur*, state which) _____. When Avery *et al.* treated the III*S* extract with **proteolytic** enzymes trypsin and chymotrypsin, transformation of II*R* (*occurred* or *failed to occur*, state which)_____. When Avery *et al.* treated the III*S* extract with **ribonuclease** (RNase), transformation of II*R* (*occurred* or *failed to occur*, state which)_____. When Avery *et al.* treated the III*S* extract with **deoxyribonuclease** (DNase), transformation of II*R* (*occurred* or *failed to occur*, state which)_____.

(c) Hershey and Chase infected one culture of *Estherichia coli* with ^{35}S-labeled phage and another culture with ^{32}P-labeled phage after which they agitated the infected cells in blenders to shear the attached phages from the bacterial cell surfaces. After centrifugation, bacterial cells are expected to be in the (**supernatant** or **pellet**, state which)_____, while the sheared-off phages are expected in the (*supernatant* or *pellet*, state which)_____. Radioactivity counts of the ^{35}S-labeled culture would be expected to be highest in the (*supernatant* or *pellet*, state which)_____ if DNA is the genetic material, while such counts in the ^{32}P-labeled culture would be expected to be highest in the (*supernatant* or *pellet*, state which)_____ if DNA is the genetic material.

(d) Below is the mutation frequency and **absorption spectrum** of bacteria plotted against **ultraviolet** wavelength and the ultraviolet absorption spectra of nucleic acids and proteins. What conclusion may be drawn from these data?

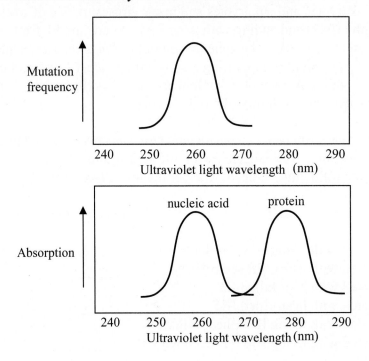

(e) Below is a table of DNA content (in picograms) in two types of cells (*n* = sperm, *2n* = red blood precursor cells).* How do these data support the hypothesis that DNA is the genetic material? Why would such support be considered *indirect* rather than *direct*?

Organism	*n*	*2n*
Human	3.25	7.30
Chicken	1.26	2.49
Trout	2.67	5.79
Carp	1.65	3.49
Shad	0.91	1.97

*Data from Klug and Cummings, *Concepts of Genetics*, 8th ed.

Concepts/Processes in Question 1: Two major lines of evidence indicate that DNA is the genetic material: **transformation** and **differential labeling.**

Analysis of Question 1:

Level 1. Review the work of Griffith (1927) Avery, MacLeod, and McCarty (1944), and Hershey and Chase (1952) before attempting this question.

General background information to orient student to the issues addressed in the questions below

Two lines of direct evidence and two lines of indirect evidence indicated that DNA is the genetic material in prokaryotes and eukaryotes and many viruses. A line of work beginning with Griffith (1927) and ending with Avery, MacLeod, and McCarty (1944) supported the hypothesis that DNA is the genetic material in *Pneumococci,* while Hershey and Chase (1952) provided supporting results with phage T2. Indirect evidence came from comparisons of DNA content in haploid and diploid cells and the mutagenesis spectrum generated by exposure to ultraviolet light.

This is the classic setup with the Griffith experiment --- injection provides an assay for transformation

(a) Griffith discovered that *Streptococcus pneumonia* (*Pneumococci*) caused pneumonia in mice.[1] In his experiments, mice were injected with different strains of treated and untreated bacteria.[2] For each of the following, indicate whether the mice *lived* or *died*.[3]

<u>*lived* or *died*?</u>

(1) mice injected with living III*S* (virulent)   _____
(2) mice injected with living II*R* (avirulent)   _____
(3) mice injected with heat-killed II*R*   _____
(4) mice injected with heat-killed III*S*   _____
(5) mice injected with living II*R* + heat-killed III*S*   _____
(6) mice injected with living III*S* + heat-killed II*R*   _____

Sentence 1: Critical to Griffith's work is the finding that *Pneumococci* cause pneumonia when injected.

Sentence 2: Life or death of the injected mouse sets up the assay system for transformation. If mice are injected with III*S* (**virulent**) bacteria, they die. If injected with II*R* (**avirulent**) bacteria, they live.

Sentence 3 and answers: Heat kills and therefore renders bacteria harmless. Consider that some component of III*S* can be transferred to II*R* to make II*R* virulent.

lived **or** *died*?

(1) mice injected with living III*S* (virulent)

Mouse dies because the bacteria cause pneumonia.

(2) mice injected with living II*R* (avirulent)

Mouse lives because the II*R* strain does not cause pneumonia.

(3) mice injected with heat-killed II*R*

Mouse lives for two reasons: first, II*R* does not cause pneumonia and second, bacteria are heat-killed.

(4) mice injected with heat-killed III*S*

Mouse lives because, even though living III*S* is virulent, it is heat-killed and can not cause pneumonia.

(5) mice injected with living II*R* + heat-killed III*S*

Mouse dies. This is the critical part of the experiment and demonstrates the presence of a transforming principle. Because the III*S* bacteria are heat-killed, they can't kill the mouse (see #4 above), and II*R* can't kill the mouse, either (see # 2 above). Since the mouse dies, something must have conferred virulence on the living II*R* bacteria. Transformation has occurred, in that some agent (transforming factor) from the heat-killed III*S* strain rendered *IIR* virulent.

(6) mice injected with living *IIIS* + heat-killed *IIR*

Mouse dies because of living III*S* bacteria.

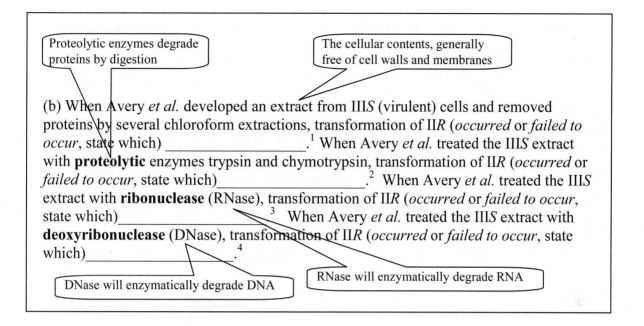

Proteolytic enzymes degrade proteins by digestion

The cellular contents, generally free of cell walls and membranes

(b) When Avery *et al.* developed an extract from III*S* (virulent) cells and removed proteins by several chloroform extractions, transformation of II*R* (*occurred* or *failed to occur*, state which) _____.[1] When Avery *et al.* treated the III*S* extract with **proteolytic** enzymes trypsin and chymotrypsin, transformation of II*R* (*occurred* or *failed to occur*, state which)_____.[2] When Avery *et al.* treated the III*S* extract with **ribonuclease** (RNase), transformation of II*R* (*occurred* or *failed to occur*, state which)_____[3] When Avery *et al.* treated the III*S* extract with **deoxyribonuclease** (DNase), transformation of II*R* (*occurred* or *failed to occur*, state which)_____.[4]

DNase will enzymatically degrade DNA

RNase will enzymatically degrade RNA

Sentence 1 and answer: Given a complex mixture of cellular components (proteins, RNA, DNA, etc.) the idea was to individually remove each so as to determine the nature of Griffith's transforming factor. Removal of proteins by chloroform extraction did not halt transformation, so transformation *occurred* (DNA was still intact).

Sentence 2 and answer: Same answer as in Sentence 1 except that the proteins were removed with trypsin and chymotrypsin. Removal of proteins by such enzymes did not halt transformation, so transformation *occurred* (DNA was still intact).

Sentence 3 and answer: Removal of RNA by RNase did not halt transformation, so transformation *occurred* (DNA was still intact).

Sentence 4 and answer: Removal of DNA by DNase stoped transformation, so transformation *failed,* (DNA levels were mostly degraded so as to effectively halt transformation). Since transformation no longer occurs after selective removal of DNA and since virulence is a hereditary trait in *Pneumococci*, DNA must be the hereditary material in such organisms.

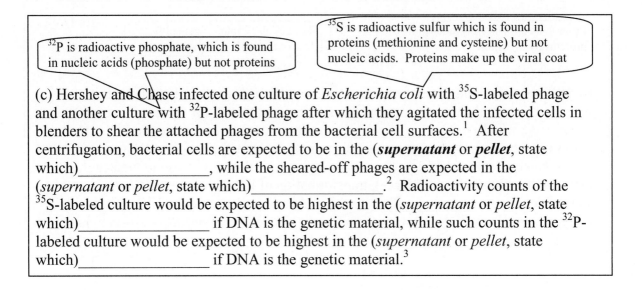

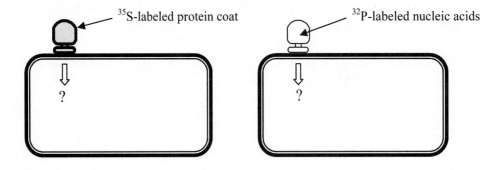

Sentence 1: Picture two separate cultures set up with one culture infected with ^{35}S-labeled phage and the other infected with ^{32}P-labeled phage. Phage are attached to the outside of the bacteria and are most likely injecting their genetic material into the bacteria. It would seem more logical to assume that whatever is injected is the genetic material, as opposed to what remains on the outside of the bacterial cell. The question is: what is injected, the protein (labeled with ^{35}S) or the nucleic acid (labeled with ^{32}P)? So how do you determine what is injected? Agitation will shear off whatever is left on the exterior of each bacterium.

Sentence 2 and answer: Since bacterial cells are larger, centrifugation will *pellet* the them but leave whatever has been sheared from the cell surface in the *supernatant*.

Sentence 3 and answer: If the genetic material is protein, then the centrifuged tube containing the ^{35}S-labeled phage will be radioactive in the pellet because it contains whatever was injected into the bacterial cell. If the genetic material is nucleic acid, then the centrifuged tube containing the ^{32}P-labeled phage will be radioactive in the pellet. Since DNA is the genetic material and it is a nucleic acid, the pellet from the culture infected with the ^{32}P-labeled phage, when agitated and centrifuged, was determined to be radioactive. So radioactivity counts in supernatant of the ^{35}S-labeled culture would be expected to be highest in the (*supernatant* or *pellet*, state which) - __*supernatant*__ if DNA is the genetic material, while such counts in the ^{32}P-labeled culture would be expected to be highest in the (*supernatant* or *pellet*, state which)__*pellet*__ if DNA is the genetic material.

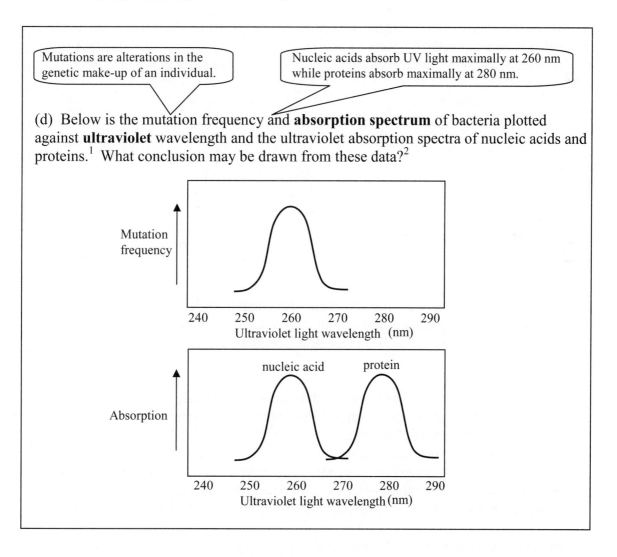

> Mutations are alterations in the genetic make-up of an individual.

> Nucleic acids absorb UV light maximally at 260 nm while proteins absorb maximally at 280 nm.

(d) Below is the mutation frequency and **absorption spectrum** of bacteria plotted against **ultraviolet** wavelength and the ultraviolet absorption spectra of nucleic acids and proteins.[1] What conclusion may be drawn from these data?[2]

Sentence 1: The overall idea behind comparing **UV absorbance** with mutation frequency is based on the likelihood that whatever wavelength causes the most mutations (hereditary alterations) will probably align with the material that absorbs the most energy from UV light.

Sentence 2 and answer: Since the mutation maximum clearly coincides with the absorption maximum of nucleic acid, proteins are likely excluded from being the genetic material. This is indirect evidence (perhaps coincidental) that DNA is the genetic material.

Some red blood cells lack nuclei but precursor cells typically contain nuclei and are usually $2n$.

(e) Below is a table of DNA content (in picograms) in two types of cells (n = sperm, $2n$ = red blood precursor cells)*.[1] How do these data support the hypothesis that DNA is the genetic material?[2] Why would such support be considered *indirect* rather than *direct*?[3]

Organism	n	$2n$
Human	3.25	7.30
Chicken	1.26	2.49
Trout	2.67	5.79
Carp	1.65	3.49
Shad	0.91	1.97

*Data from Klug and Cummings, *Concepts of Genetics*, 8th ed.

Sentence 1: Cells that contain n nuclei would have half as many chromosomes as cells that contain $2n$ nuclei. Since chromosomes were known to carry the hereditary determiners (as of about 1915), there would be half as many chromosomes in the n cells compared to the $2n$ cells.

Sentence 2 and answer: Since **eukaryotic** chromosomes are made of both DNA and protein, one would expect that whatever substance is the genetic material should be half as abundant in an n cell as compared with a $2n$ cell. The data in the table show that DNA fits that expectation. However, since chromosomes are also made of proteins, proteins fit that expectation, also. But proteins in each whole cell would not exist in a 1:2 ratio. This, along with the information in parts (a) through (d) in this question, shows that DNA is consistent with being the genetic material.

Sentence 3 and answer: As stated above, eukaryotic chromosomes are composed of both DNA and protein, so the data in part (e) are not conclusive. It could be coincidental that DNA content in an n cell is half that in a $2n$ cell. Thus, the data are consistent with DNA being the genetic material but not conclusive. We may say that these data provide indirect evidence that DNA is the genetic material.

(a) There are a number of common terms and expressions that characterize the genetic material in both prokaryotes and eukaryotes. Of the choices below, select the single choice that is most accurate.

    A. DNA, single stranded, antiparallel, $(A+G)/(T+U) = 1.0$
    B. RNA, double stranded, parallel, $(A+G)/(T+U) = 1.0$
    C. DNA, double stranded, antiparallel, $(A+G)/(T+C) = 1.0$
    D. DNA, double stranded, antiparallel, $(A+T)/(G+C) = 1.0$
    E. DNA, double stranded, antiparallel, $(A+G)/(T+C) = $ variable
    F. DNA, double stranded, parallel, $(A+T)/(G+C) = $ variable

(b) Below is a table listing the approximate base compositions of two viruses. What conclusions, concerning the nature of viral nucleic acids, can be reached from these data?

	C	A	G	U
Influenza A (H0N1)	23.6	23.3	21.2	31.8

	C	A	G	T
Herpes simplex (HSV-1)	33.4	16.3	33.6	16.7

Concepts/Processes in Question 2: This question addresses base **complementarity**, **RNA**, **DNA**, and **data interpretation**.

Analysis of Question 2:

> Both prokaryotes and eukaryotes have DNA as their genetic material

Level 2. (a) There are a number of common terms and expressions that characterize the genetic material in both prokaryotes and eukaryotes.[1] Of the choices below, select the single choice that is most accurate.[2]

    A. DNA, single stranded, antiparallel, $(A+G)/(T+U) = 1.0$
    B. RNA, double stranded, parallel, $(A+G)/(T+U) = 1.0$
    C. DNA, double stranded, antiparallel, $(A+G)/(T+C) = 1.0$
    D. DNA, double stranded, antiparallel, $(A+T)/(G+C) = 1.0$
    E. DNA, double stranded, antiparallel, $(A+G)/(T+C) = $ variable
    F. DNA, double stranded, parallel, $(A+T)/(G+C) = $ variable

Sentence 1: The question centers on nonviral organisms identified as prokaryotic (bacteria) and eukaryotic --- both of which have double-stranded DNA as their genetic material.

Sentence 2 and answer: As mentioned above, all prokaryotic and eukaryotic genomes are double stranded and DNA. Because all DNAs are antiparallel in their makeup, the only issue left is the ratio. In double-stranded DNA, the ratio of **purines** (adenine and guanine) to **pyrimidines** (thymine and cytosine) should be 1.00. In addition, since A pairs with T and G pairs with C, the (A + G)/(T + C) ratio must also be 1.00. The answer is choice C.

> Considerable molecular variety in viral genomes; see below

(b) Below is a table listing the approximate base compositions of two viruses.[1] What conclusions concerning the nature of viral nucleic acids can be reached from these data?[2]

	C	A	G	U
Influenza A (H0N1)	23.6	23.3	21.2	31.8

	C	A	G	T
Herpes simplex (HSV-1)	33.4	16.3	33.6	16.7

Sentence 1: Viral genomes can exist in a number of different configurations: DNA, RNA, single stranded, double stranded, linear, and circular.

Sentence 2 and answer: Clues are offered in the table in that U (uracil) is seen in *Infuenza A* and T (thymine) is seen in *Herpes simplex*. Therefore one can immediately say that *Influenza* is an RNA virus, while *Herpes simplex* is a DNA virus. As for single- or double-strandedness, notice that the **purine/pyrimidine ratio** for *Influenza A* is not unity and that there is not a quantitative relationship between A and U. Based on this information, one may conclude that *Influenza* is a single-stranded RNA virus. Notice that for *Herpes simplex*, the purine/pyrimidine ratio is about 1.0 (16.3 + 33.6)/(33.4 + 16.7) = 1.004. In addition, notice that the A and T amounts are quite similar, as are the G and C amounts. These data are consistent with, but do not prove, the fact that the DNA of *Herpes simplex* is double stranded. Given these data, it is not possible to determine whether the DNA or RNA genomes are linear or circular.

Question 3: Level 3

(a) To the right is a shorthand sketch of a dinucleotide. Does it represent DNA or RNA? Is the star closest to the 5' or 3' (state which) end of this **dinucleotide**? Suppose that the phosphate identified by the arrow was radioactive (^{32}P). Suppose also that the dinucleotide was cleaved with an enzyme (spleen diesterase, for example) that breaks the covalent bonds connecting the phosphates to the 5' carbons. After cleavage with this enzyme, to which base would the phosphate now be attached, C or T?

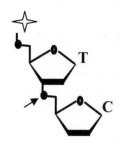

(b) Assume that the following single strand of DNA was used as a template for the synthesis of a strand of RNA, and the innermost phosphate (the one directly attached to the 5' carbon of the ribose sugar) of all the UTPs was labeled with ^{32}P.

3'-CGAATTAGTGAG-5'

Assume also that the newly synthesized RNA strand was degraded to completion by an enzyme that cleaves RNA only at the covalent bond that connects the 5' carbon of the sugar to the phosphate. Which of the resulting nucleotide(s) would you expect to now carry the ^{32}P?

Concepts/Processes in Question 3: The critical issues of **nucleic acid structure**, **5'-3' polarity**, and **complementarity** are presented.

Analysis of Question 3:

> This issue is critical to understanding the structure and function of nucleic acids.

> A dinucleotide is two nucleotides covalently linked 5'-3'.

Level 3: (a) To the right is a shorthand sketch of a dinucleotide.[1] Does it represent DNA or RNA?[2] Is the star closest to the 5' or 3' (state which) end of this **dinucleotide**?[3] Suppose that the phosphate identified by the arrow was radioactive (^{32}P).[4] Suppose also that the dinucleotide was cleaved with an enzyme (spleen diesterase, for example) that breaks the covalent bonds connecting the phosphates to the 5' carbons.[5] After cleavage with this enzyme, to which base would the phosphate now be attached, C or T?[6]

> Enzymes will cut nucleic acids at different places. See below for more information for a sketch.

Sentence 1: The sketch is a typical shorthand that is useful for many questions dealing with nucleic acid structure and function. See the general orientations below:

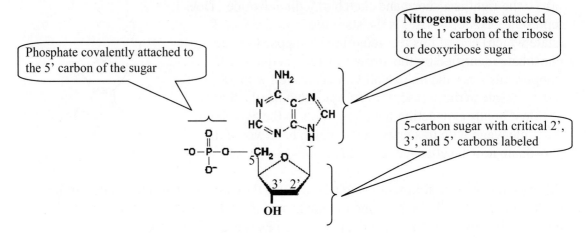

When two nucleotides are connected to make a dinucleotide, a 5'-3' **phosphodiester linkage** is created (with the elimination of water), as shown below.

Sentence 2 and answer: Since the figure in the original question contains a T for thymine, it must be a DNA dinucleotide because RNA does not contain thymine; it contains uracil (U) in its place.

Sentence 3 and answer: Consider the structure presented above and relate it to the following figure given in the original problem. Notice that the star is at the 5' carbon side; therefore, the star is at the 5' end of the dinucleotide.

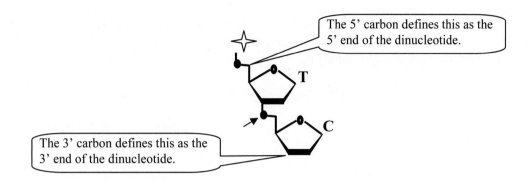

The 5' carbon defines this as the 5' end of the dinucleotide.

The 3' carbon defines this as the 3' end of the dinucleotide.

Sentence 4: The ^{32}P originated from the innermost phosphate of a nucleoside triphosphate (ATP, GTP, CTP, or TTP). It was originally attached to the 5' carbon of the nucleoside triphosphate.

Sentences 5 and 6 and answer: Notice that after cleavage, the phosphate (^{32}P in this case) that was attached to the 5' carbon of the cytosine nucleotide, is now attached to the 3' carbon of the nucleotide in the 5' direction. So in this case the T nucleotide would contain the ^{32}P after cleavage with spleen diesterase.

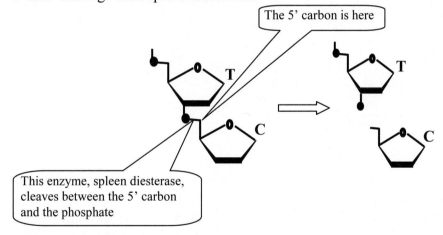

The 5' carbon is here

This enzyme, spleen diesterase, cleaves between the 5' carbon and the phosphate

A complementary strand will be synthesized in the 5'-3' direction, copying this strand from the 3' to the 5' end

(b) Assume that the following single strand of DNA was used as a template for the synthesis of a strand of RNA, and the innermost phosphate (the one directly attached to the 5' carbon of the ribose sugar) of all the UTPs was labeled with ^{32}P.[1]

3'-CGAATTAGTGAG-5'

This enzyme will cut the RNA between the 5'carbon and the phosphate, transferring the labeled phosphate to the 3' carbon of the 5' neighbor.

Assume also that the newly synthesized RNA strand was degraded to completion by an enzyme that cleaves RNA only at the covalent bond that connects the 5' carbon of the sugar to the phosphate.[2] Which of the resulting nucleotide(s) would you expect to now carry the ^{32}P?[3]

Sentence 1: A complementary strand is to be synthesized, and it will be an RNA strand with a labeled UTP entering the synthesized stand. The new strand will be built from the 5'-3' direction, copying the given strand in the 3'-5' direction, as shown below (incorporated uracils are underlined):

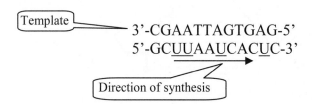

Template — 3'-CGAATTAGTGAG-5'
5'-GCUUAAUCACUC-3'
Direction of synthesis

Sentences 2 and 3 and answer: Re-read Sentences 5 and 6 in part (a) of this question and notice that with this type of enzymatic cleavage, the original 5'-labeled phosphate is transferred to the 3' carbon of the 5' neighbor. In that case, the C, U, and C bases will now be attached to the ^{32}P:

3'-CGAATTAGTGAG-5'
5'-GCUUAAUCACUC-3'

Question 4: Level 3

(a) When double-stranded DNA is heated sufficiently, the duplex separates into single strands (**denaturation** or **melting**). As shown by monitoring UV absorbance during strand separation, a hyperchromic shift occurs in which the Abs_{260} of single-stranded structures is (*more* or *less*, state which) _____ than that of double-stranded structures. In addition, the amount of energy (heat) needed to denature DNA is influenced by GC content. Given the figure below and assuming all strands are of equal length, which melting profile is likely to represent DNA with the highest GC content, the *solid* line or *dotted* line?[4]

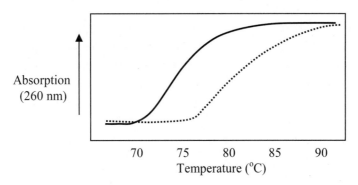

Absorption (260 nm)

70   75   80   85   90

Temperature ($^{\circ}$C)

(b) Phage lambda (λ) is a double-stranded DNA (48,502 base pairs) bacteriophage with a linear chromosome when packaged in the phage protein coat. Assume that a mutant strain ($\lambda\Delta$) was created by removal (a deletion) of 12,000 base pairs in the approximate center of the λ chromosome. Assume also that a mixture of λ and $\lambda\Delta$ DNA was mixed, heated to 95 $^{\circ}$C for 10, minutes and slowly cooled to 20 $^{\circ}$C to allow the strands to reanneal (reform duplexes). The figures below represent **homoduplexes** (both strands $\lambda\Delta$ DNA or both strands λ DNA) and **heteroduplexes** (one λ and one $\lambda\Delta$ strand). Using the symbols $\lambda\Delta$, λ, or $\lambda\lambda\Delta$, identify each strand below.

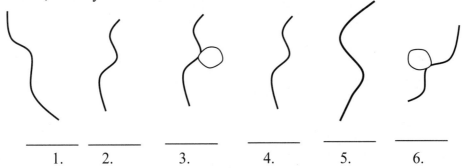

1.   2.   3.   4.   5.   6.

(c) The point at which 50% of a denaturing DNA (or RNA) sample is single stranded is called the melting temperature (T_m). For sequences longer than 14 bases (on one strand), it is approximated using the following equation

$$T_m = 64.9 + 41 \times \frac{(nG + nC - 16.4)}{N}$$

where nG and nC are the number of guanine and cytosine nucleotides respectively and N is the total number of nucleotides in the annealing strand. From the above equation, would you expect the T_m to *increase* or *decrease* as the GC content of the annealing strand increases? Explain your answer.

(d) Assume that in a 0.9M NaCl solution, the T_m for a given DNA sample is 83 °C. Would you expect the T_m to *increase* or *decrease* in a 0.0009M NaCl solution? Explain your answer.

Concepts/Processes in Question 4: This question addresses the phenomena of the **hyperchromic shift, denaturation, annealing, T_m, and data interpretation.**

Analysis of Question 4:

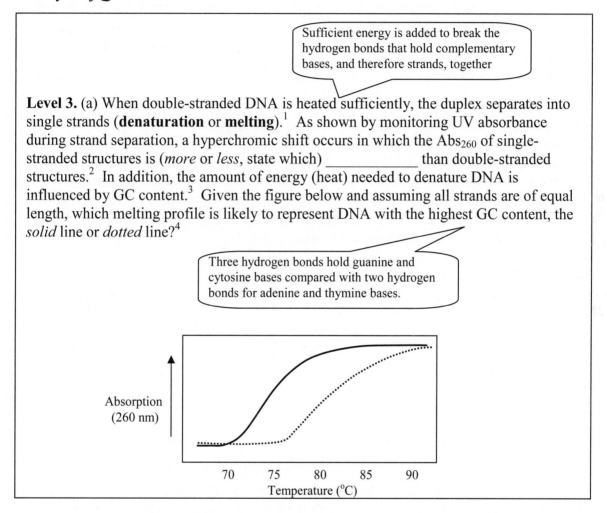

> Sufficient energy is added to break the hydrogen bonds that hold complementary bases, and therefore strands, together

Level 3. (a) When double-stranded DNA is heated sufficiently, the duplex separates into single strands (**denaturation** or **melting**).[1] As shown by monitoring UV absorbance during strand separation, a hyperchromic shift occurs in which the Abs_{260} of single-stranded structures is (*more* or *less*, state which) _____ than double-stranded structures.[2] In addition, the amount of energy (heat) needed to denature DNA is influenced by GC content.[3] Given the figure below and assuming all strands are of equal length, which melting profile is likely to represent DNA with the highest GC content, the *solid* line or *dotted* line?[4]

> Three hydrogen bonds hold guanine and cytosine bases compared with two hydrogen bonds for adenine and thymine bases.

Sentence 1: Heat denatures or melts nucleic acids because hydrogen bonds holding GC and AT(U) bases together are more readily broken as the energy (heat) increases to a temperature beyond about 70° C.

Sentence 2 and answer: Single stranded nucleic acids absorb more energy at 260 nm than double stranded nucleic acids. Therefore, as nucleic acids go from double stranded to single stranded, *more* absorbance (at 260 nm) occurs.

Sentence 3: When guanine (G) and cytosine (C) form complementary pairs, three hydrogen bonds are formed. With adenine (A) and thymine (T) two hydrogen bonds are formed. As the number of hydrogen bonds increases, the energy (heat) needed to separate complementary pairs increases.

Sentence 4 and answer: On the abscissa temperature in °C is plotted, while on the ordinate one sees Abs$_{260}$, which, by increasing, is indicating the transition from double to single stranded nucleic acids. The position of the dotted line indicates that more heat is needed to affect the separation; therefore, the dotted line contains the highest percentage of GC pairs.

> Both λ and λΔ will be in the mixture, which, when heated, should be composed of long and relatively short (3/4 as long) single-stranded stretches of DNA

(b) Phage lambda (λ) is a double-stranded DNA (48,502 base pairs) bacteriophage with a linear chromosome when packaged in the phage protein coat.[1] Assume that a mutant strain (λΔ) was created by removal (a deletion) of 12,000 base pairs in the approximate center of the λ chromosome.[2] Assume also that a mixture of λ and λΔ DNA was mixed, heated to 95 °C for 10 minutes, and slowly cooled to 20 °C to allow the strands to reanneal (reform duplexes).[3] The figures below represent **homoduplexes** (both strands λΔ DNA or both strands λ DNA) and **heteroduplexes** (one λ and one λΔ strand). Using the symbols λΔ, λ, or λλΔ, identify each strand below.[4]

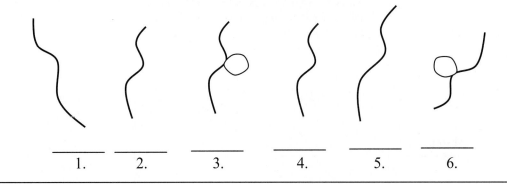

1. _____   2. _____   3. _____   4. _____   5. _____   6. _____

Sentences 1 and 2: Consider that two populations of phage chromosomes are being referred to here. One has 48,502 base pairs, and another is missing 12,000 base pairs from the center. The chromosome with the deletion (λΔ) will be about ¾ the length of the non-deleted chromosome (λ).

Sentence 3: When the double-stranded structures are heated to 95 °C for 10 minutes, they denature so that complementary single strands are produced. As the mixture is cooled to 20 °C, complementary strands unite and double-stranded structures are again formed. Since all the strands are from the same genome (one intact and the other carrying a deletion), all the single strands should eventually form double strands except where a heteroduplex is formed. In such cases a single-stranded "loop" should occur, and it should be in the approximate middle of the chromosome.

Sentence 4 and answers: The longest strand, without the loop, should be where the complementary strands of λ reannealed, while the shortest strand, without the loop, should be where the complementary strands of λΔ reannealed. Where there is a loop, a λΔ strand has reannealed with a λ strand. The answers are as follows:

1. λ   2. λΔ   3. λλΔ   4. λΔ   5. λ   6. λλΔ

> There are many equations that have been developed, some sophisticated, to estimate T_m. Equations generally differ as a function of strand length and ionic concentration

(c) The point at which 50% of a denaturing DNA (or RNA) sample is single stranded is called the melting temperature (T_m). For sequences longer than 14 bases (on one strand), it is approximated using the following equation:

> Look carefully at this equation and note that %GC and overall length of the strands are the only variables

$$T_m = 64.9 + 41 \times \frac{(nG + nC - 16.4)}{N}$$

where nG and nC are the number of guanine and cytosine nucleotides respectively and N is the total number of nucleotides in the annealing strand.[1] From the above equation, would you expect the T_m to *increase* or *decrease* as the GC content of the annealing strand increases?[2] Explain your answer.[3]

Sentence 1: This sentence sets the background for the question by providing one of many T_m equations that have been developed. Merely looking at the equation shows that as the number of GC pairs increases, T_m increases.

Sentences 2 and 3, and answers: As mentioned above, the T_m increases as the GC content of the annealing strand increases. This is because there are three hydrogen bonds holding GC pairs together, compared with two H bonds for AT pairs.

> Sodium ions (Na^+) will interact with the negative charges on the phosphates along the nucleic acid backbone

(d) Assume that in a 0.9M NaCl solution, the T_m for a given DNA sample is 83 °C.[1] Would you expect the T_m to *increase* or *decrease* in a 0.0009M NaCl solution?[2] Explain your answer.[3]

Sentence 1: Picture a number of negative charges on the nucleic acid backbone interacting with the positively charged Na^+. The molarity given is 0.9M, so there should be an abundance of Na^+ present compared to 0.0009M described in the next sentence. A T_m of 83 °C would be the temperature at which half of the sample is single stranded and half is double stranded.

Sentences 2 and 3 and answers: As the salt concentration decreases from 0.9M to 0.0009M, the amount of shielding of the negative (repulsive) charges on phosphates decreases. As that shielding decreases, repulsion between the negative charges on the phosphates on complementary strands increases, pushing the strands apart and making the helix less stable. So, with a reduction in Na^+, the T_m should be lower because the double helix is less stable and more susceptible to denaturation by heat.

Question 5: Level 2

Assume that a bacterial culture is grown on medium containing radioactive thymine (^{3}H-T) until essentially all of the thymine in the DNA is radioactive. Assume also that the ^{3}H-T-labeled bacteria were washed and transferred to a medium containing nonradioactive thymine for one round of replication (approximately 22 minutes). Given the double-stranded sequences below (1-4), which one is likely to represent the replicated double-stranded structure? (Note: A, T, G, C represent typical nucleotides, and ^{3}T represents labeled thymine.)

	1	**2**	**3**	**4**
One strand:	AG^{3}TC	AG^{3}TC	AG^{3}TC	AG^{3}TC
Other strand:	AGTC	TCAG	UC^{3}AG	^{3}TCAG

Concepts/Processes in Question 5: This question addresses **DNA replication**, **polarity restrictions**, and **applications**.

Analysis of Question 5:

> Thymine should be incorporated opposite adenine..

> Assume **semiconservative** replication.

Level 2. Assume that a bacterial culture is grown on medium containing radioactive thymine (^{3}H-T) until essentially all of the thymine in the DNA is radioactive.[1] Assume also that the ^{3}H-T-labeled bacteria were washed and transferred to a medium containing nonradioactive thymine for one round of replication (approximately 22 minutes).[2] Given the doublestranded sequences below (1-4), which one is likely to represent the replicated double-stranded structure?[3] (Note: A, T, G, C represent typical nucleotides, and ^{3}T represents labeled thymine.)

	1	2	3	4
One strand:	AG^{3}TC	AG^{3}TC	AG^{3}TC	AG^{3}TC
Other strand:	AGTC	TCAG	UC^{3}AG	^{3}TCAG

Sentence 1: When bacteria are grown on radioactive medium, they will take up nutrients from the medium and incorporate them into their own structures.

Sentence 2: After one round of semiconservative replication in a nonlabeled medium, each daughter strand will be composed of one ^{3}H-T-labeled strand and one unlabeled strand:

Sentence 3 and answer: Given that the complementary strand will be composed of AT and GC pairs and one strand should have the ^{3}H label and the other should not, choice 2 seems most appropriate.

A strain of *E. coli* was grown for many generations in ^{15}N (present in the form of NH_4Cl), a heavy isotope of nitrogen (^{14}N). Assume that such "density-labeled" DNA has a density of 1.73 g/cm^3 ($H_2O = 1.00$ g/cm^3). Assume that DNA containing only the common form of nitrogen, ^{14}N, has a density of 1.71 g/cm^3. Bacteria from the fully labeled ^{15}N culture were washed and transferred to ^{14}N medium for one generation. DNA was extracted (call this generation 1) and its density determined by ultracentrifugation. Bacteria were also allowed to undergo another generation in ^{14}N and DNA was extracted (call this generation 2).

(a) Under a semiconservative scheme of replication, what would be the expected density (or densities) of extracted double-stranded DNA from generation 1? Under a semiconservative scheme of replication, what would be the expected density (or densities) of extracted double-stranded DNA from generation 2?

(b) Under a **conservative** scheme of replication, what would be the expected density (or densities) of the extracted double-stranded DNA from generation 1? Under a conservative scheme of replication, what would be the expected density (or densities) of the extracted double-stranded DNA from generation 2?

(c) Under a **dispersive** scheme of replication, what would be the expected density (or densities) of the extracted double-stranded DNA from generation 1? Under a dispersive scheme of replication what would be the expected density (or densities) of the extracted double-stranded DNA from generation 2?

(d) One of scientists' concerns when interpreting the classic experiment of Meselson and Stahl was that the hybrid-density DNA, instead of being composed of one heavy, ^{15}N-containing strand and one light, ^{14}N-containing strand in generation 1, was really an aggregate of strands that just happen to have a hybrid density. To address this concern, Meselson and Stahl heated hybrid-density DNA to 100 $^{\circ}C$, cooled it quickly to inhibit reannealing, and re-centrifuged. If the hybrid-density DNA from generation 1 was as predicted by a semiconservative model, how many distinct bands and what proportions of each would Meselson and Stahl observe after such treatment?

(e) Assuming that the **molar percentage** of adenine in the generation 1 DNA sample in part (a) was 30%, what would be the expected molar percentages of the other nitrogenous bases in this double stranded DNA?[1] Would your answers change for the generation 2 DNA sample?[2]

Concepts/Processes in Question 6: This question illustrates models of **DNA replication**, **density labeling**, and **experimental design**.

Analysis of Question 6:

> Nitrogen is a component of the nitrogenous bases, adenine, guanine, cytosine, and thymine in DNA.

Level 3. A strain of *E. coli* was grown for many generations in ^{15}N (present in the form of NH_4Cl), a heavy isotope of nitrogen (^{14}N).[1] Assume that such "density-labeled" DNA has a density of 1.73 g/cm^3 (H_2O = 1.00 g/cm^3).[2] Assume that DNA containing only the common form of nitrogen, ^{14}N, has a density of 1.71 g/cm^3.[3] Bacteria from the fully labeled ^{15}N culture were washed and transferred to ^{14}N medium for one generation.[4] DNA was extracted (call this generation 1) and its density determined by ultracentrifugation.[5] Bacteria were also allowed to undergo another generation in ^{14}N and DNA was extracted (call this generation 2).[6]

> Ultracentrifugation will allow the separation of ^{15}N-containing DNA from DNA containing the common form of ^{14}N

Sentence 1: If a strain of *E. coli* is grown for many generations in a particular nutrient, ^{15}N in this case, that nitrogen becomes incorporated in a variety of molecules including DNA. It is the nitrogenous bases in DNA that pick up the ^{15}N. Eventually, after many generations, most of the ^{14}N is replaced by ^{15}N and is thus "density-labeled" DNA.

Sentence 2: Since the density-labeled DNA has a density of 1.73 g/cm^3 it can be distinguished by ultracentrifugation from DNA with different densities.

Sentences 3 and 4: If the original density-labeled bacteria were washed and transferred to ^{14}N medium for one generation, then the DNA should pick up ^{14}N bases as the DNA is replicating. Generation 1 bacteria will have replicated once in ^{14}N medium.

Sentence 5: Ultracentrifugation will allow separation of heavy, hybrid, and light DNA based on the different densities generated by the use of ^{15}N.

Sentence 6: DNA from bacteria that have passed through two rounds (generation 2) of replication in ^{14}N medium will be centrifuged to determine the presence and perhaps distribution of ^{14}N and ^{15}N. The general model for semiconservative replication is given below:

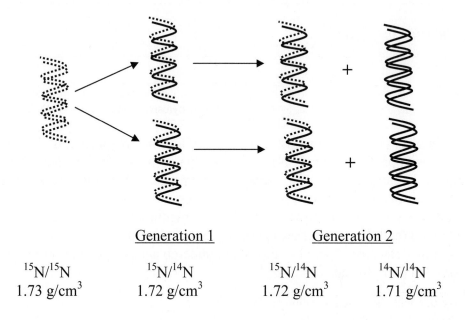

	Generation 1		Generation 2	
^{15}N/^{15}N	^{15}N/^{14}N		^{15}N/^{14}N	^{14}N/^{14}N
1.73 g/cm^3	1.72 g/cm^3		1.72 g/cm^3	1.71 g/cm^3

(a) Under a semiconservative scheme of replication, what would be the expected density (or densities) of extracted double-stranded DNA from generation 1?[1] Under a semiconservative scheme of replication, what would be the expected density (or densities) of extracted double-stranded DNA from generation 2?[2]

Sentence 1 and answer: After one round of semiconservative replication in ^{14}N medium, each DNA duplex would be composed of one heavy and one light strand for a density of 1.72 g/cm^3.

Sentence 2 and answer: After two rounds of semiconservative replication in ^{14}N medium, there would be two populations of DNA: one population composed of one heavy and one light strand for a density of 1.72 g/cm^3 and the other population composed of both light strands for a density of 1.71 g/cm^3.

(b) Under a **conservative** scheme of replication, what would be the expected density (or densities) of the extracted double-stranded DNA from generation 1?[1] Under a conservative scheme of replication, what would be the expected density (or densities) of the extracted double-stranded DNA from generation 2?[2]

Sentences 1 and 2 and answers: Under a conservative scheme, the original stand remains intact, while the copied strand is completely new. See the figure below for an explanation.

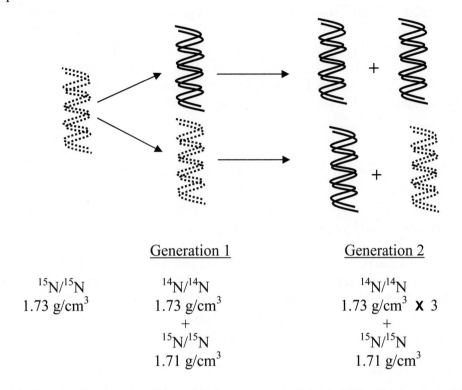

Generation 1

Generation 2

$^{15}N/^{15}N$
1.73 g/cm³

$^{14}N/^{14}N$
1.73 g/cm³
+
$^{15}N/^{15}N$
1.71 g/cm³

$^{14}N/^{14}N$
1.73 g/cm³ **X** 3
+
$^{15}N/^{15}N$
1.71 g/cm³

(c) Under a **dispersive** scheme of replication, what would be the expected density (or densities) of the extracted double-stranded DNA from generation 1?[1] Under a dispersive scheme of replication what would be the expected density (or densities) of the extracted double-stranded DNA from generation 2?[2]

Sentence 1 and answer: Under a dispersive scheme of replication, depending on how one configures the breakup of the strands, each daughter strand would be composed of intermittent ^{15}N and ^{14}N DNA single strands joined by complementary base pairing. The density of the generation 1 DNAs would therefore be intermediate or 1.72 g/cm³.

Sentence 2 and answer: Since the ^{14}N would be added to the 1.72 g/cm³ DNA from generation 1, one would expect a "washing out" of the ^{15}N density as another equivalent of ^{14}N is added. Therefore, in generation 2 there would be again one population with a density of $(1.72 + 1.71)/2 = 1.715$ g/cm³.

(d) One of scientists' concerns when interpreting the classic experiment of Meselson and Stahl was that the hybrid-density DNA, instead of being composed of one heavy, ^{15}N-containing strand and one light, ^{14}N-containing strand in generation 1, was really an aggregate of strands that just happen to have a hybrid density.[1] To address this concern, Meselson and Stahl heated hybrid-density DNA to 100 °C, cooled it quickly to inhibit reannealing, and re-centrifuged.[2] If the hybrid-density DNA from generation 1 was as predicted by a semiconservative model, how many distinct bands and what proportions of each would Meselson and Stahl observe after such treatment?[3]

Sentence 1: The hybrid-density DNA predicted by the semiconservative model would have precisely equal amounts of ^{15}N-single-stranded DNA and ^{14}N-single-stranded DNA held together by hydrogen bonds. Aggregates might have varying amounts of each and not be associated by hydrogen bonds.

Sentence 2 and 3 and answers: The semiconservative scheme of replication predicts that in generation 1, the two strands (heavy and light) would be held together by hydrogen bonding. When such bonds are broken by 100° C, and the mixture is cooled quickly, the strands remain separate. Centrifugation should produce equal amounts of the heavy and light strands; therefore, two bands would be seen.

(e) Assuming that the **molar percentage** of adenine in the generation 1 DNA sample in part (a) was 30%, what would be the expected molar percentages of the other nitrogenous bases in this double stranded DNA?[1] Would your answers change for the generation 2 DNA sample?[2]

Sentence 1 and answer: Since A and T occur in equal amounts and G and C occur in equal amounts in double stranded structures, there would be 30% T and 40% divided by two for G and C. So, G and C would each equal 20%.

Sentence 2 and answer: Since the base pairing rules remain constant from one double helix to another, there should be no difference in the percentages of bases in subsequent generations.

Question 7: Level 3

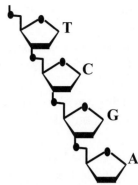

To the right is a figure depicting a polymer of four nucleotides.

(a) Do the sugars in this molecule each contain *five* or *six* carbons? Are the sugars *ribose* or *deoxyribose*? Is there an OH group attached to the 2' carbon of these sugars?

(b) Assume that the molecule depicted in the figure served as a template for a newly synthesized DNA strand composed of four nucleotides. What would be the expected base sequence and polarity of the newly synthesized DNA? Fill in the blank spaces provided below for the newly synthesized strand:

$$5' -\underline{\quad}-\underline{\quad}-\underline{\quad}-\underline{\quad}-3'$$

(c) Assume that one of the precursors for the newly synthesized DNA strand was a ^{32}P-labeled (innermost phosphate) guanine nucleoside triphosphate. Given that spleen diesterase cleaves the covalent bond between the phosphate and the 5' carbon of a DNA polymer, which nucleotide would be expected to contain the ^{32}P after cleavage with spleen diesterase? On what carbon will the ^{32}P now be attached?

Concepts/Processes in Question 7: This question centers on **DNA structure**, **complementarity**, and **polarity**.

Analysis of Question 7:

Level 3. To the right is a figure depicting a polymer of four nucleotides.[1]

(a) Do the sugars in this molecule each contain *five* or *six* carbons?[2] Are the sugars *ribose* or *deoxyribose*?[3] Is there an OH group attached to the 2' carbon of these sugars?[4]

Sentence 1: Notice that the four nucleotides are connected in typical phosphodiester linkages and thymine is present. This indicates that the strand is a DNA and the sugars are deoxyribose.

Sentence 2 and answer: Since the strand is a nucleic acid and nucleic acids contain either ribose or deoxyribose as their sugars, there must be five carbons in each sugar.

Sentence 3 and answer: Since thymine (T) is one of the bases, the strand must be a DNA strand; therefore, the sugar must be a deoxyribose.

Sentence 4 and answer: Since the sugars are deoxyribose, there must be no OH group attached to the 2' carbon.

> Important: the focus has now shifted to the newly synthesized strand, which is an **antiparallel** complement of the strand pictured above

(b) Assume that the molecule depicted in the figure served as a template for a newly synthesized DNA strand composed of four nucleotides.[5] What would be the expected base sequence and polarity of the newly synthesized DNA?[6] Fill in the blank spaces provided below for the newly synthesized strand:

5' -___-___-___-___-3'

Sentence 5: Since the strand in the figure is serving as a template for the newly synthesized strand, two issues must be addressed: base complementation and polarity.

Sentence 6 and answer: Since the original strand is DNA and the complementary strand is also DNA, there will be no uracil present and all the rules of complementarity will be standard. The 5' end is identified by noting which end has a 5' carbon. Notice that the top of the figure shows a 5' carbon attached to a phosphate. In addition, the antiparallel nature of the strands will give the following answer:

5' -_T_-_C_-_G_-_A_-3'

(c) Assume that one of the precursors for the newly synthesized DNA strand was a ^{32}P-labeled (innermost phosphate) guanine nucleoside triphosphate.[7] Given that spleen diesterase cleaves the covalent bond between the phosphate and the 5' carbon of a DNA polymer, which nucleotide would be expected to contain the ^{32}P after cleavage with spleen diesterase?[8] On what carbon will the ^{32}P now be attached?[9]

Sentence 7: Since all precursors to nucleic acid synthesis are made up of 5' dNTPs, the ^{32}P would be donated from the 5' carbon of dGTP.

Sentences 8 and 9 and answer: Spleen diesterase will cleave the bond between the ^{32}P on the 5' carbon of the guanine nucleotide and transfer it to the 3' carbon of its 5' neighbor, which is C in this case (see below at the arrow to the right).

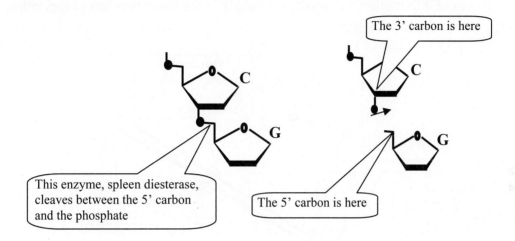

The sketch below is of a short section of DNA (not drawn to scale) of a **prokaryotic** chromosome in the process of replication.   Boxes pointing to various structures request specific pieces of information that you are to supply in the corresponding spaces below.

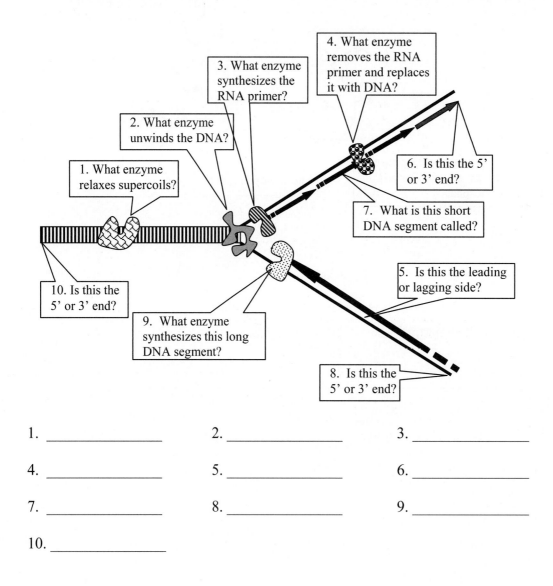

1. _____

2. _____

3. _____

4. _____

5. _____

6. _____

7. _____

8. _____

9. _____

10. _____

Concepts/Processes in Question 8: This question examines the process and **enzymology** of **DNA replication.**

Analysis of Question 8:

Critical aspects of replication include antipolarity, complementarity, and enzymology.

Level 3. The sketch below is of a short section of DNA (not drawn to scale) of a **prokaryotic** chromosome in the process of replication.[1] Boxes pointing to various structures request specific pieces of information that you are to supply in the corresponding spaces below.[2]

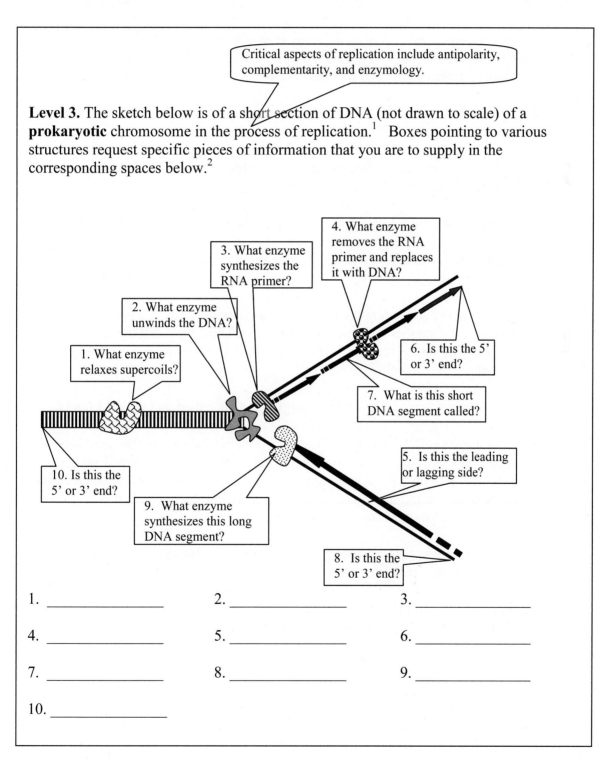

4. What enzyme removes the RNA primer and replaces it with DNA?

3. What enzyme synthesizes the RNA primer?

2. What enzyme unwinds the DNA?

1. What enzyme relaxes supercoils?

6. Is this the 5' or 3' end?

7. What is this short DNA segment called?

5. Is this the leading or lagging side?

10. Is this the 5' or 3' end?

9. What enzyme synthesizes this long DNA segment?

8. Is this the 5' or 3' end?

1. _____   2. _____   3. _____

4. _____   5. _____   6. _____

7. _____   8. _____   9. _____

10. _____

Sentence 1: This is a typical **replication fork** that is opening from right to left. In other words, the original strands of the double helix are opening as the fork proceeds from right to left. It is important to consider polarity of strands and enzymes involved in answering this question.

Sentence 2 and answers: The information requested is critical in understanding the nature of DNA replication. Below are answers and explanations for each component.

1. Because **supercoils** occur as the helix is unwound, an enzyme, a **topoisomerase** called *DNA gyrase*, reverses the supercoils and allows the helix to continue to unwind and open for replication.

2. A group of proteins, collectively called **helicases**, opens and destabilizes the helix.

3. An RNA polymerase, called **primase,** provides the free 3'-OH upon which DNA polymerization is dependent.

4. **DNA polymerase I** removes the RNA primer and replaces it with DNA.

5. Since synthesis is continuous on the side referred to, it is called the **leading strand.**

6. Notice that the arrow points to the end of a strand that has just been synthesized. All synthesis of nucleic acids is 5'-3', meaning that the last nucleotide to be added is at the 3' end. Therefore, the pointer is at the *3' end* of the strand.

7. Each short section of DNA on the **lagging side** is called an **Okazaki fragment**.

8. There are several ways to tackle this question, but the easiest way is to look at the direction of synthesis of the complementary strand. As mentioned several times above, all synthesis of nucleic acids is 5'-3', therefore making the end of the complementary strand the 5' end. If the complementary strand's end is 5', then the strand at the pointer is the *3' end.*

9. **DNA polymerase III** is the enzyme that typically synthesizes the long continuous strands of DNA.

10. Follow the strand from the pointer to the other end on the right. In Question #8, that was the 3' end. Therefore, pointer #10 identifies the *5' end.*

Assume that you are microscopically examining mitotic metaphase cells of an organism with a 2n chromosome number of 4 (one pair **metacentric** and one pair **acrocentric**). Assume also that the cell passed through one S phase of radioactive labeling (^{3}H-thymidine) just prior to the period of observation at metaphase. You observe the following (dots represent locations of radioactive decay and the location of label):

(a) Of the three modes of DNA replication (conservative, dispersive, and semiconservative), which, if any, can be eliminated as a mode of DNA replication from this information? (More than one answer may be used if appropriate.)

(b) Assume that a second experiment was performed, and after the first passage of an S phase in the presence of ^{3}H-thymidine, the cells were allowed to complete a single mitosis but were then washed and transferred to a medium with nonradioactive thymidine and examined at the subsequent metaphase. Such chromosomes had the following labeling pattern. Based on information in parts (a) and (b), of the three modes of DNA replication (conservative, dispersive, and semiconservative), which, if any, can be eliminated as a mode of DNA replication from this information? (More than one answer may be used if appropriate.)

(c) Based on information from parts (a) and (b) above, and focusing your attention on the labeled chromatids from part (a), what would be the labeling pattern of the DNA strands within each labeled chromatid (*pattern A*, *pattern B*, *neither*, or *either*)? (Dotted lines represent a labeled strand of DNA; solid lines represent nonlabeled DNA.)

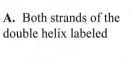

A. Both strands of the double helix labeled

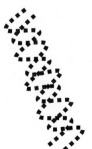

B. One strand of the double helix labeled

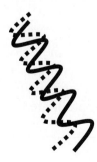

(d) Based on information from parts (a) and (b), and focusing your attention on the labeled chromatids from part (b), what would be the labeling pattern of the DNA strands within each labeled chromatid (*pattern A*, *pattern B*, *neither*, or *either*)? (Dotted lines represent a labeled strand of DNA; solid lines represent nonlabeled DNA.)

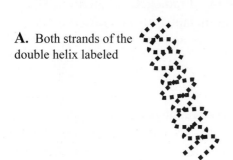

A. Both strands of the double helix labeled

B. One strand of the double helix labeled

Concepts/Processes in Question 9: This problem illustrates **DNA replication** in **eukaryotes** and stresses **experimental design** associated with a demonstration of **semiconservative replication**.

Analysis of Question 9:

Each mitotic spread should have four chromosomes with eight chromatids total

Metacentric chromosomes have the centromere in the middle while acrocentric chromosomes have the centromere off center

Level 4: Assume that you are microscopically examining mitotic metaphase cells of an organism with a *2n* chromosome number of 4 (one pair **metacentric** and one pair **acrocentric**).[1] Assume also that the cell passed through one S phase of radioactive labeling (^{3}H-thymidine) just prior to the period of observation at metaphase.[2] You observe the following (dots represent locations of radioactive decay and the location of label):[3]

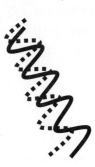

(a) Of the three modes of DNA replication (conservative, dispersive, and semiconservative), which, if any, can be eliminated as a mode of DNA replication from this information?[4] (More than one answer may be used if appropriate.)

Sentence 1: Metaphase chromosomes are most visible because they are condensed and readily stain. With a *2n* chromosome number of 4, there should be four chromosomes visible, each with chromatids, for eight chromatids total. Metacentric chromosomes will have an approximately equal arm ratio (chromatids extending from the centromere at about equal lengths), while in acrocentric chromosomes, one arm will be slightly shorter than the other.

Sentence 2: During the S phase, chromosomes replicate and in doing so will pick up the ^{3}H-thymidine, which is complementary to adenine. Only those chromosomes that have passed through the S phase will be labeled.

Sentence 3: Notice that there are the expected four chromosomes and that each chromatid is labeled.

Sentence 4 and answer: Given the completion of an S phase in ^{3}H-thymidine, each original unlabeled double helix now picks up label on complementary strands under a semiconservative model. Let the broken line represent ^{3}H-thymidine-labeled DNA and the solid line represent unlabeled DNA. At the chromosomal level, the significant, but only, difference between the replication pattern in prokaryotes and that in eukaryotes is that the products of replication are held together by a **centromere** in eukaryotes but not in prokaryotes. Looking at the three representations below, and comparing them to the results presented in the metaphase chromosomes above shows that the *conservative* model can be eliminated. Dotted lines represent ^{3}H-labeled DNA.

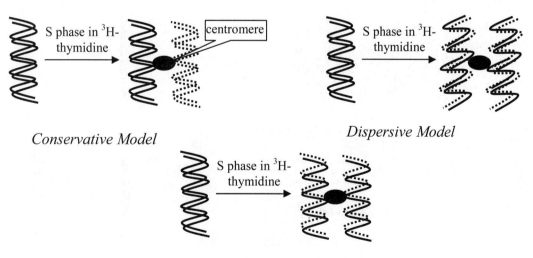

Conservative Model

Dispersive Model

Semiconservative Model

(b) Assume that a second experiment was performed, and after the first passage of an S phase in the presence of ^{3}H-thymidine, the cells were allowed to complete a single mitosis but were then washed and transferred to a medium with nonradioactive thymidine and examined at the subsequent metaphase.[5] Such chromosomes had the following labeling pattern.[6] Based on information in parts (a) and (b), of the three modes of DNA replication (conservative, dispersive, and semiconservative), which, if any, can be eliminated as a mode of DNA replication from this information?[7] (More than one answer may be used if appropriate.)

Sentences 5, 6, and 7 and answer: After the first round of replication in the ^{3}H-thymidine, the chromosomes would have the pattern (see below) as indicated in the original problem. Each chromatid is labeled, and under a semiconservative model, each DNA helix is half labeled as in the figures described in Sentence 4 above. If one replicates each chromosome in unlabeled medium the following DNA labeling pattern would be observed. Each chromosome would have one labeled chromatid (each DNA helix half labeled) and one unlabeled chromatid, as indicated below. The labeling patterns described in parts (a) and (b) are consistent with a semiconservative model.

The conservative model was eliminated by information given in part (a) and the *dispersive model* can be eliminated by information given in part (b) because in the dispersive model, both chromatids of each chromosome would retain label, albeit diluted.

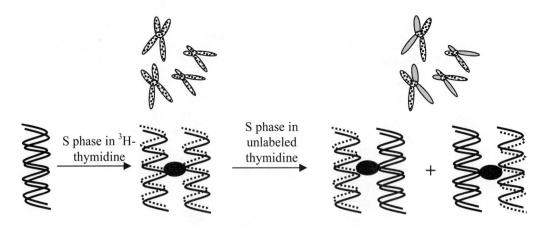

Semiconservative Model

(c) Based on information from parts (a) and (b), and focusing your attention on the labeled chromatids from part (a), what would be the labeling pattern of the DNA strands within each labeled chromatid (*pattern A*, *pattern B*, *neither*, or *either*.)?[8] (Dotted lines represent a labeled strand of DNA; solid lines represent nonlabeled DNA.)

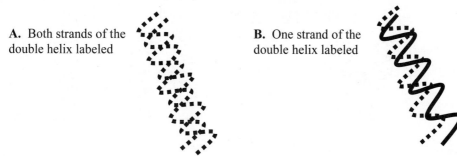

A. Both strands of the double helix labeled

B. One strand of the double helix labeled

Sentence 8 and answer: Notice in the figure below that each chromatid after one round of replication in label contains DNA in which one strand is labeled and the other is unlabeled. The answer is therefore B.

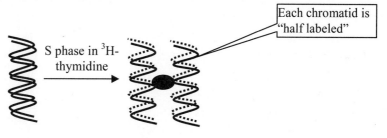

S phase in ^{3}H-thymidine

Each chromatid is "half labeled"

Semiconservative Model

(d) Based on information from parts (a) and (b), and focusing your attention on the labeled chromatids from part (b), what would be the labeling pattern of the DNA strands within each labeled chromatid (*pattern A*, *pattern B*, *neither*, or *either*)?[9] (Dotted lines represent a labeled strand of DNA; solid lines represent nonlabeled DNA.)

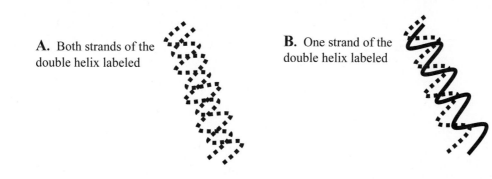

A. Both strands of the double helix labeled

B. One strand of the double helix labeled

Sentence 9 and answer: Again, notice in the figure below that each labeled chromatid after two rounds of replication (one round in label and the second free of label) contains DNA in which one strand is labeled and the other is unlabeled. The answer is therefore B.

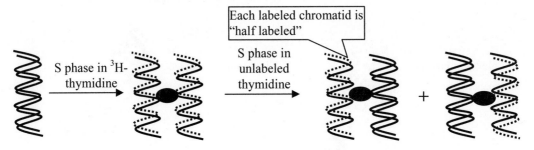

Semiconservative Model

Session VI

Molecular Biology: Techniques and Analytical Approaches

Concepts/Processes	Level(s)	Relevant Question(s)	Page(s)
Restriction digestion, electrophoresis	2	1	137
Restriction digestion, mapping	2	2	139
Polymerase chain reaction	3	3	144
DNA sequencing	4	4	148

Question 1: Level 2

Assume that you have a **plasmid** with the following **restriction enzyme** digestion sites labeled *EcoRI* and *HindIII* and that the overall size of the plasmid is 4000 base pairs. Focusing your attention on Gel A, in what lane, 1-5, is a likely electrophoretic pattern resulting from complete digestion of this plasmid with the *EcoRI* enzyme? Focusing your attention on Gel B, in what lane (1-5) is a likely electrophoretic pattern resulting from complete digestion of this plasmid with the *HindIII* enzyme?

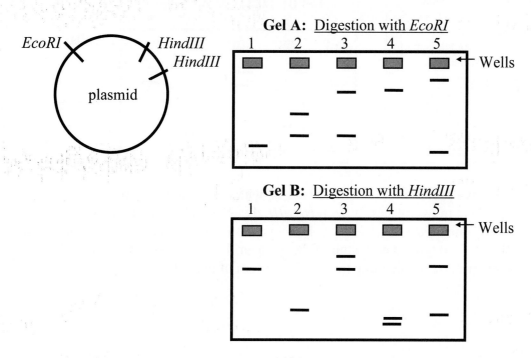

Concepts/Processes in Question 1: This problem addresses basic methods in molecular biology: **restriction digestion** and **electrophoresis.**

Analysis of Question 1:

Plasmids are composed of circular, double-stranded DNA of varying sizes

Restriction enzymes used in this question cut double-stranded DNA at specific places defined by base sequence

Level 2: Assume that you have a **plasmid** with the following **restriction enzyme** digestion sites labeled *EcoRI* and *HindIII* and that the overall size of the plasmid is 4000 base pairs.[1] Focusing your attention on Gel A, in what lane, 1-5, is a likely electrophoretic pattern resulting from complete digestion of this plasmid with the *EcoRI* enzyme?[2] Focusing your attention on Gel B, in what lane (1-5) is a likely electrophoretic pattern resulting from complete digestion of this plasmid with the *HindIII* enzyme?[3]

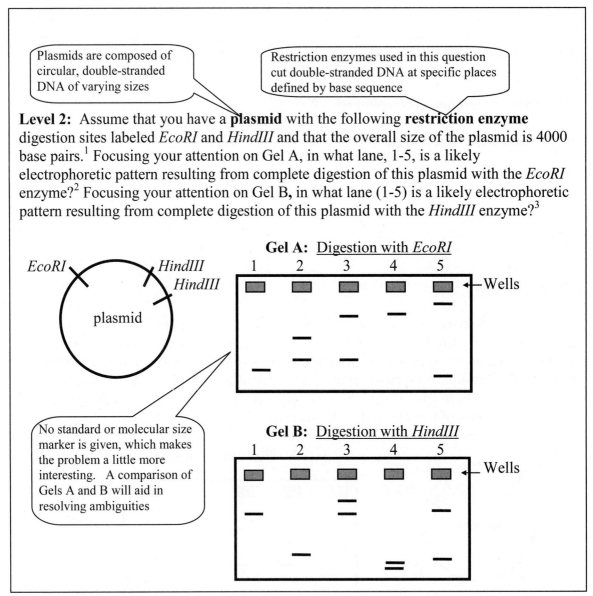

No standard or molecular size marker is given, which makes the problem a little more interesting. A comparison of Gels A and B will aid in resolving ambiguities

Sentence 1: If a plasmid is cut in one place, as with *EcoRI*, there should be one large product. If cut in two places, as with *HindIII*, there should be one relatively large product and one quite small product. During electrophoresis, large fragments migrate more slowly (and remain at the top of the gel near the wells) compared to small fragments, which migrate more toward the bottom of the gel.

Sentence 2 and answer: With no molecular size markers (typically used in gels), the problem takes on a little ambiguity. However, in Gel A, we should be looking for a single fragment remaining quite close to the well because it is large (one cut). Notice that in *lane 4*, there is one fragment close to the well that is probably the correct choice. Examination of Gel B supports this conclusion, because the slow-migrating band in lane 5 is high in the gel and indicates a large fragment, slightly smaller than the one in lane 4 of Gel A.

Sentence 3 and answer: In Gel B, we should be looking for two fragments, one relatively large and one quite small. In *lane 5*, there are two fragments, one migrating slowly (large) and one migrating farther down the gel.

Question 2: Level 2

Restriction sites play an important role in gene mapping and diagnostics because they provide, among other things, heritable chromosomal reference points. Establishing the location of such sites, restriction mapping, is often accomplished by examining fragments formed by single and double digestion of DNA with restriction enzymes. Below is a representation of an agarose gel containing a typical size marker (λ DNA digested with *HindIII*), the uncut linear fragment, the fragment digested with *EcoRI*, and the fragment digested with *PstI*.

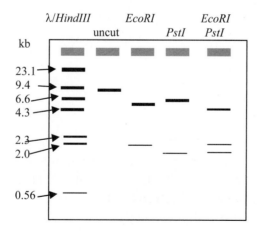

(a) What is the approximate size of the uncut fragment?

   A. 23 kilobases
   B. 18 kilobases
   C. 8 kilobases
   D. 4 kilobases
   E. insufficient information to answer this question

(b) Why do the bands near the bottom of the gel seem to be lighter in stain intensity than those at the top?

(c) Which of the figures below represents the correct relative positions of the *EcoRI* and *PstI* restrictions?

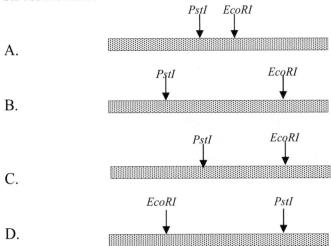

Concepts/Processes in Question 2: This problem addresses an analysis of **agarose gel electrophoresis** as it applies to the development of a **restriction map**. Included is an analysis of **DNA migration patterns** as they relate to a **molecular size standard** (λ/*HindIII*) and **staining intensity**.

Analysis of Question 2:

Restriction sites are locations where restriction enzymes cut DNA

Double digestion is accomplished by using two restriction enzymes at the same time

Level 2: Restriction sites play an important role in gene mapping and diagnostics because they provide, among other things, heritable chromosomal reference points.[1] Establishing the location of such sites, restriction mapping, is often accomplished by examining fragments formed by single and double digestion of DNA with restriction enzymes.[2] Below is a representation of an agarose gel containing a typical size marker (λ DNA digested with *HindIII*), an uncut linear fragment, the fragment digested with *EcoRI*, and the fragment digested with *PstI*.[3]

A size marker allows you to estimate the length, in kilobase pairs (kb), of a separated sample of DNA

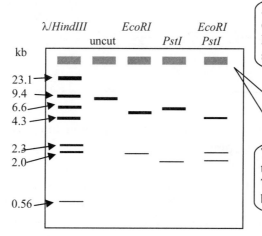

These are the wells where the DNA sample is placed. The largest fragments will be closest to the wells

(a) What is the approximate size of the uncut fragment?[4]

    A. 23 kb
    B. 18 kb
    C. 8 kb
    D. 4 kb
    E. insufficient information to answer this question

(b) Why do the bands near the bottom of the gel seem to be lighter in stain intensity than those at the top?[5]

(c) Which of the figures below represents the correct relative positions of the *EcoRI* and *PstI* restrictions? [6]

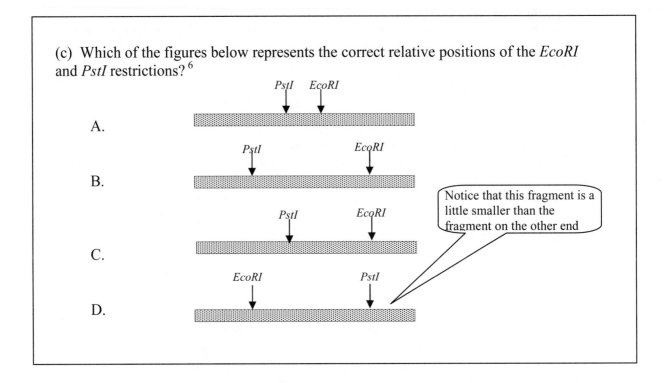

Sentence 1: This is a background sentence giving you some idea of the significance and use of restriction mapping.

Sentence 2: A restriction enzyme such as *EcoRI* cuts a section of DNA into pieces, depending on how many *EcoRI* restriction sites are present in the target DNA. Double digests help in the construction of the restriction map because they identify fragments that are divisible because they have other restriction sites. This will be clearer as the analysis proceeds.

Sentence 3: A typical agarose gel is composed of a "marker" lane with known DNA sized fragments. Often the lambda (λ = a bacteriophage) chromosome cut with *HindIII* is used. Note the sizes of fragments listed on the left side of the gel. The bands one sees are linear; therefore, one can only compare linear fragments to such a size standard.

Sentence 4 and answer: To determine the approximate size of a fragment on the gel, compare the distance traveled to the λ/*HindIII* standard. Such an approach is a little deceiving because separation of nucleic acids on agarose gels follows a log scale, with the separation between larger fragments much less dramatic than the separation between smaller fragments at the bottom of the gel. Notice that the uncut fragment is slightly lower in the gel than the 9.4 kb band in the λ/*HindIII* standard. Of the choices given in the answers, 8 kilobases seems like a good approximation. The answer is therefore C.

Sentence 5 and answer: Consider that the smaller fragments travel the fastest and are therefore at the bottom of the gel. Smaller fragments take up less stain and therefore appear fainter than the larger fragments at the top of the gel. Theoretically, each band has the same number of fragments for a given sample.

Sentence 6 and answer: The single digest with *EcoRI* gives two fragments, one around 6 kb and the other around 2 kb. Digestion with *PstI* gives two fragments also, one about 6.5 kb and the other about 1.5 kb. In the double digest, notice that the 6 kb band from the *EcoRI* digest has been fragmented, and you are left with what appear to be 4.5 kb, 2.0 kb, and 1.5 kb fragments. One can envision two models that alter the position of the *PstI* site with reference to the *EcoRI* site:

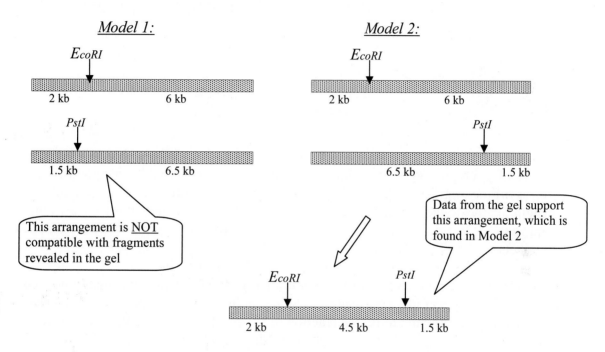

Question 3: Level 3

The polymerase chain reaction (PCR) allows researchers a method of amplifying a section of DNA without using traditional cloning of fragments in plasmids. Generally, three temperatures are used in a typical PCR: 94-96 °C, 50-65 °C, and 72 °C.

(a) Given the following double-stranded structure, sketch what is occurring during the temperatures mentioned above. Be certain to indicate the 5'-3' orientations of all nucleic acids in your sketch.

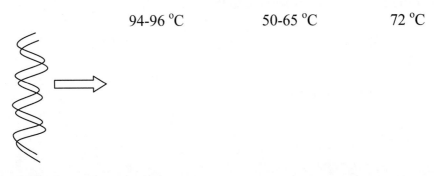

(b) During a typical PCR, two populations of products are formed. One population forms off the original DNA strands of amplification and is often long and variable in length relative to the subsequent products, while all the subsequent products are uniform and usually shorter in length. Explain, in diagram form, the origin of different-sized PCR products.

(c) Assume that when examining results from a typical PCR, the investigator noticed that instead of a single product being amplified, multiple, nonspecific products were also amplified. In an attempt to rid the reaction of nonspecific products, the investigator tried the following actions. Which would you consider the most likely remedy? Why?

    A. decrease the denaturation temperature
    B. increase the denaturation temperature
    C. decrease the annealing temperature
    D. increase the annealing temperature
    E. increase the concentration of primer
    F. increase the concentration of dNTPs
    G. decrease the extension temperature

Concepts/Processes in Question 3: This question addresses the **polymerase chain reaction,** including **annealing**, **polarity**, and **complementarity**.

Analysis of Question 3:

> These temperatures can vary depending on the condition of the template and primer

> Billions of copies of a DNA section can be made if certain parameters are known

Level 3. The polymerase chain reaction (PCR) allows researchers a method of amplifying a section of DNA without using traditional cloning of fragments in plasmids.[1] Generally, three temperatures are used in a typical PCR: 94-96 °C, 50-65 °C, and 72 °C.[2] (a) Given the following double-stranded structure, sketch what is occurring during the temperatures mentioned above.[3] Be certain to indicate the 5'-3' orientations of all nucleic acids in your sketch.[4]

| 94-96 °C | 50-65 °C | 72 °C |

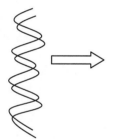

Sentence 1: Given information on the sequence of the desired fragment or sequences flanking the desired fragment, in the presence of a heat-stable polymerase, sufficient amplification of a fragment can be easily accomplished.

Sentence 2: The three temperatures used in a typical PCR are designed to denature the target DNA (highest temperature), anneal the primers by base hybridization (lowest temperature), and extend the primers by a heat-stable DNA polymerase (middle temperature, around 72°C.). Slight variations of a degree or two can occur for the denaturation and extention steps, and significant variations in the annealing temperature can occur based on the length and base content of the primers.

Sentences 3 and 4 and answers: Below is a description of the general events in a PCR. The primers are indicated as short dotted lines. Notice the 5' and 3' polarity orientations as the primers associate with the target sequences.

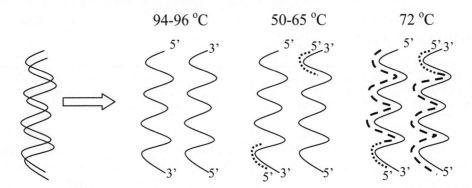

(b) During a typical PCR, two populations of products are formed. One population forms off the original DNA strands of amplification and is often long and variable in length relative to the subsequent products, while all the subsequent products are uniform and usually shorter in length.[5] Explain, in diagram form, the origin of different-sized PCR products.[6]

Sentences 5 and 6 and answer: The primers originally bind to the DNA at the sites first exposed by denaturation. At the extension step, those primers are extended until either the time of the cycle ends (usually between 30 and 90 seconds) or polymerase fails for one reason or another. Therefore, the length of the first two amplification products for a given helix is variable. However, once the first two products are made for a given helix, the products provide the primer annealing sites for subsequent amplifications, as shown below.

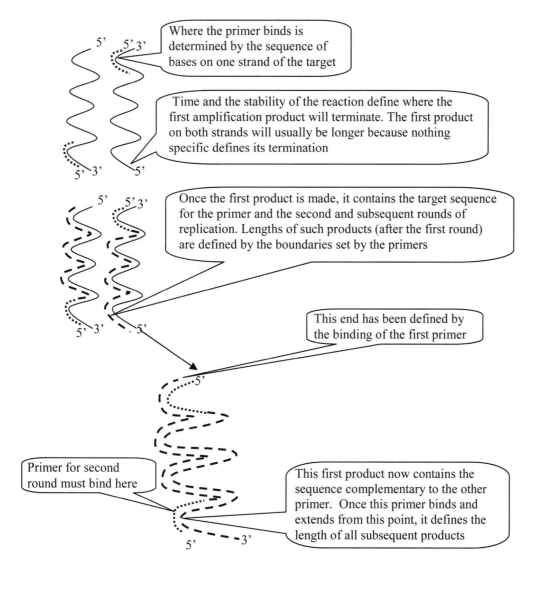

(c) Assume that when examining results from a typical PCR, an investigator noticed that instead of a single product being amplified, multiple, nonspecific products were also amplified.[7] In an attempt to rid the reaction of nonspecific products, the investigator tried the following actions.[8] Which would you consider the most likely remedy?[9] Why?

    A. decrease the denaturation temperature
    B. increase the denaturation temperature
    C. decrease the annealing temperature
    D. increase the annealing temperature
    E. increase the concentration of primer
    F. increase the concentration of dNTPs
    G. decrease the extension temperature

Sentence 7: It often happens in a PCR that nonspecific products are formed, for which there may be a variety of explanations, including primers that are impure, too concentrated, or too short, complex and variable targets, and poorly constructed environment (buffers, Mg^{2+} concentration, and too low an annealing temperature).

Sentences 8 and 9 and answer: Of the factors listed, the easiest and most likely solution is choice D because slight increases in the annealing temperature will decrease nonspecific binding and may decrease the amplification of nonspecific products.

Question 4: Level 4

DNA sequencing using the Sanger method involves annealing a 5'-end labeled (*) oligonucleotide (primer) to a single-stranded piece of DNA to be sequenced. The primer is designed so that its 3' end is adjacent to the section to be sequenced (target). Theoretically, four different reactions are set up, each containing the four normal nucleotide precursors to DNA (dATP, dTTP, dCTP, and dGTP) and a different ddNTP (**dideoxynucleotide**) to serve as a chain terminator. (A more efficient adaptation of this procedure replaces the 5'-end labeling primer with a different fluorescent dye on each ddNTP so that one, rather than four, reaction is needed). Once the DNA polymerizing enzyme is added, products of different lengths are separated on a **polyacrylamide** gel and the sequence is determined, given that the sequence on the gel is complementary to the sequence on the DNA of interest.

(a) Sketch the normal arrangement of a single-stranded DNA target and 5'-end labeled primer.

(b) What is the critical difference between a dATP and a ddATP in terms of structure of the nucleotide and function in DNA sequencing?[7]

(c) Assume that the sequence of the following target DNA was desired:

3'-CGATTCGATT-5'

Given the figure below, sketch in a banding pattern that is consistent with the desired sequence.

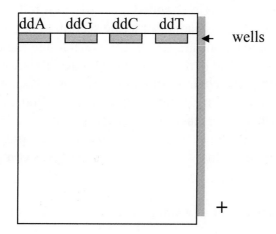

(d) Generally, the concentration of a given ddNTP is about 1/100 the concentration of its dNTP counterpart. Assume that a new investigator miscalculated the ddNTP concentration and used 1/1000 instead of 1/100. What influence would you expect this mishap to have on the distribution of bands on the gel?

Concepts/Processes in Question 4: DNA sequencing, end-labeling, and **gel interpretation** are examined in some detail.

Analysis of Question 4:

> Short sequence of about 10-20 bases in length

> **ddNTP** lacks a hydroxyl group on the 3' carbon and is therefore unable to support additional chain growth

Level 4. DNA sequencing using the Sanger method involves annealing a 5'-end labeled (*) oligonucleotide (primer) to a single-stranded piece of DNA to be sequenced.[1] The primer is designed so that its 3' end is adjacent to the section to be sequenced (target).[2] Theoretically, four different reactions are set up, each containing the four normal nucleotide precursors to DNA (dATP, dTTP, dCTP, and dGTP) and a different ddNTP (**dideoxynucleotide**) to serve as a chain terminator.[3] (A more efficient adaptation of this procedure replaces the 5'-end labeling primer with a different fluorescent dye on each ddNTP so that one, rather than four, reaction is needed).[4] Once the DNA polymerizing enzyme is added, products of different lengths are separated on a **polyacrylamide** gel and the sequence is determined, given that the sequence on the gel is complementary to the sequence on the DNA of interest.[5]

(a) Sketch the normal arrangement of a single-stranded DNA target and 5'-end labeled primer.[6]

Sentences 1 and 2 and answer (a): Below is a sketch of a section of DNA to be sequenced, flanked on the left (3' end) by a region complementary to the oligonucleotide primer (dotted line). The 5' end is labeled and designated with a *.

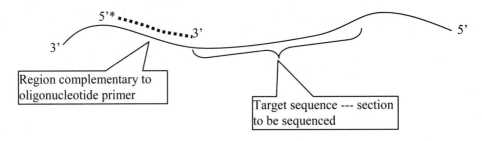

Region complementary to oligonucleotide primer

Target sequence --- section to be sequenced

(b) What is the critical difference between a dATP and a ddATP in terms of structure of the nucleotide and function in DNA sequencing?[7]

Sentences 3 and 4 and answer (b): Consider three types of nucleotides, ribonucleotide, deoxyribonucleotide, and dideoxyribonucleotide, as indicated below:

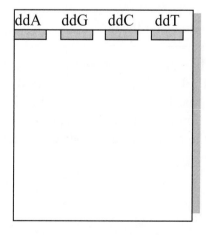

Notice the position of the arrows and focus on the presence or absence of the –OH group on the 3' and 2' carbon atoms of the ribose sugars. Since the linkage between two nucleotides in a polymer is dependent on the presence of a 3' –OH, its absence in a dideoxynucleotide would halt addition of nucleotides. Such a ddNTP can be thought of as a chain terminator. If the ddNTP had a fluorescent dye attached to it and it became the last to be incorporated in a strand, when a ddNTP is incorporated, it would not only mark each strand's length, but also mark each strand's identity (ddATP, ddTTP, ddCTP, or ddTTP).

(c) Assume that the sequence of the following target DNA was desired:

3'-CGATTCGATT-5'.

Given the figure below, sketch in a banding pattern that is consistent with the desired sequence.[8]

ddA	ddG	ddC	ddT

Sentence 5 and answer (c): The following strand would be copied with the primer binding to a sequence to the left (3' side of the target) and the newly synthesized ddNTP terminated and labeled population of strands generated as shown below:

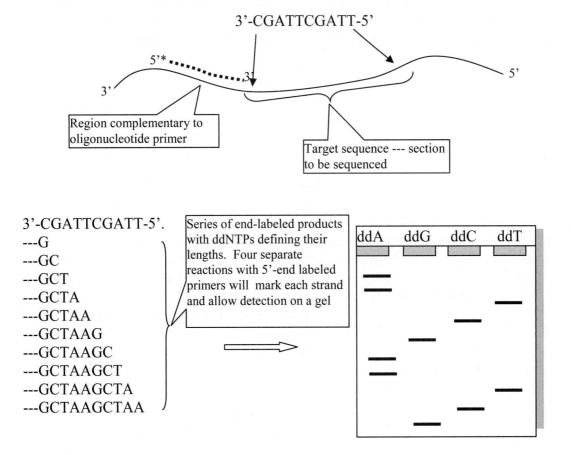

(d) Generally, the concentration of a given ddNTP is about 1/100 the concentration of its dNTP counterpart. Assume that a new investigator miscalculated the ddNTP concentration and used 1/1000 instead of 1/100. What influence would you expect this mishap to have on the distribution of bands on the gel?[9]

Sentence 9 and answer (d): Notice that the length of each strand is dependent on the random incorporation of a ddNTP. If a 10X additional dilution occurs, there would be fewer such chance incorporations, and on average, the strands would be longer. In other words, it would take longer for a ddNTP to be incorporated on average. Overall, then, one would expect the bands to run higher in the gel because they are longer.

Session VII

Molecular Biology: Pathways, Proteins, Transcription, Translation, and Mutation

Question 1: Level 1

(a) In the early 1900s, a physician named Sir Archibald Garrod found that people suffering from a particular metabolic disease, alkaptonuria, excreted abnormally large amounts of homogentisic acid in their urine.In his book *The Incidence of Alkaptonuria: A Study in Chemical Individuality*, he provided the first description of recessive inheritance in humans. Considering the relationship of genes to metabolic pathways, where would one predict that the genetic block occurs in alkaptonuria?

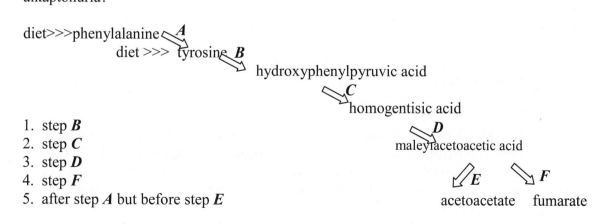

1. step *B*
2. step *C*
3. step *D*
4. step *F*
5. after step *A* but before step *E*

(b) Phenylketonuria (PKU) is a genetic disease that causes mental retardation if left untreated. It is caused by a mutant allele that behaves as an autosomal recessive. Individuals with PKU have elevated blood levels of phenylalanine and its derivatives. Considering the pathway in part (a) of this question, what steps would one reasonably consider to reduce the symptoms associated with PKU?

Concepts/Processes in Question 1: This question examines the relationship between **genotype** and **phenotype** through an analysis of **metabolic pathways**.

Analysis of Question 1:

Level 1.

> Important information here; appears as if there is a buildup of homogentisic acid in alkaptonurics

> Addresses a fundamental concept in molecular biology. Genes often influence metabolic pathways in certain ways. See discussion below

(a) In the early 1900s, a physician named Sir Archibald Garrod found that people suffering from a particular metabolic disease, alkaptonuria, excreted abnormally large amounts of homogentisic acid in their urine.[1] In his book *The Incidence of Alkaptonuria: A Study in Chemical Individuality*, he provided the first description of recessive inheritance in humans.[2] Considering the relationship of genes to metabolic pathways, where would one predict that the genetic block occurs in alkaptonuria?[3]

diet>>>phenylalanine *A*
       diet>>> tyrosine *B*
                hydroxyphenylpyruvic acid
                      C
                 homogentisic acid

1. step *B*
2. step *C*
3. step *D*   *D*
4. step *F*   maleylacetoacetic acid
5. after step *A* but before step *E*
                                 /E   *F*
                           acetoacetate   fumarate

(b) Phenylketonuria (PKU) is a genetic disease that causes mental retardation if left untreated. It is caused by a mutant allele that behaves as an autosomal recessive.[4] Individuals with PKU have elevated blood levels of phenylalanine and its derivatives.[5] Considering the pathway in part (a) of this question, what steps would one reasonably consider to reduce the symptoms associated with PKU?[6]

Sentence 1(a): There are several generalities that apply to genetically altered metabolic pathways: absence of end product, buildup of immediate precursor, and buildup of immediate precursor with impact on connecting pathways. If the enzyme at position *D* that metabolizes homogentisic acid is defective, there would be little or no maleylacetoacetic acid, with a likely buildup of the precursor homogentisic acid. Such accumulating substances often build up in the blood and eventually pass out in the urine. If one had a thorough understanding of the relationships between genes and metabolic pathways, one could say after reading Sentence 1, that the answer to the question is most likely choice 3 (step *D*).

Sentence 2(a): This sentence provides an historical perspective to the question and adds a minor, but, helpful, point. Recessive mutations that involve metabolic pathways are often "loss-of-function" and serve, when homozygous, to simply block such pathways. In the context of this question, the straightforward approach would assume that a simple metabolic block occurs at position *D*.

Sentence 3(a): Recall (see Sentence 1) the generalities that usually apply to genetically altered metabolic pathways: absence of end product, buildup of immediate precursor, and buildup of immediate precursor with impact on connecting pathways.These generalities are being referred to in the sentence that states "Considering the relationship of genes to metabolic pathways." The answer is therefore option 3, since there are no contradicting components to the question.

Sentence 4(b): Since PKU is caused by an autosomal recessive mutant allele and since phenylalanine is a member of the pathway described in the problem, it is likely that concepts applied to part (a) of the problem will also apply to part (b).

Sentence 5(b): Again, an elevated substance appears to be responsible for the phenotype. This relationship addresses the overall conceptual intent of the question.

Sentence 6(b) and answer. Since phenylalanine comes from the diet, one might attempt to counter the symptoms by reducing the intake of phenylalanine. In fact, this is the therapeutic approach to PKU. Since phenylalanine is a component of proteins, however, it can't be entirely eliminated from the diet.

Question 2: Level 2

Assume that you conduct an experiment similar to the one done by Beadle and Tatum in the 1940s that began to define the relationship between genes and chemical events in living systems. Using *Neurospora*, they provided chemical additives, call them **A**, **B**, and **C**, to minimal medium (**MM**) and scored for growth (+) or lack of growth (-). From the data in the table, (a) determine the wild-type strain, (b) construct the biochemical pathway for additives **A**, **B**, and **C**, and (c) place the mutations that define the various strains in the appropriate positions in the pathway you construct.

Strain	*MM (no additive)*	*MM+A*	*MM+B*	*MM+C*
967	-	+	+	+
q44	+	+	+	+
999	-	-	+	-
806	-	+	+	-

(a)

(b, c)

Concepts/Processes in Question 2: This question addresses the basic concepts of **gene action**, **metabolic pathway determination**, and **data interpretation**.

Analysis of Question 2:

Classic work to show that genes are involved in biochemical pathways. Mutant alleles cause blocks in metabolic pathways

This is the critical aspect of the experimental design from which the table is constructed

Level 2. Assume that you conduct an experiment similar to the one done by Beadle and Tatum in the 1940s that began to define the relationship between genes and chemical events in living systems.[1] Using *Neurospora*, they provided chemical additives, call them **A**, **B**, and **C**, to minimal medium (***MM***) and scored for growth (+) or lack of growth (-).[2] From the data in the table, (a) determine the wild-type strain, (b) construct the biochemical pathway for additives **A**, **B**, and **C**, and (c) place the mutations that define the various strains in the appropriate positions in the pathway you construct.[3]

Strain	*Control (no additive)*	*MM+A*	*MM+B*	*MM+C*
967	-	+	+	+
q44	+	+	+	+
999	-	-	+	-
806	-	+	+	-

Sentence 1: If you are unfamiliar with the Nobel-winning work of Beadle and Tatum, be certain to review it carefully. Because of its significance in illuminating the relationship between genes and chemical events within cells, its mastery is mandatory. Basically, their work led to the one-gene-one-enzyme statement.

Sentence 2: If you are unfamiliar with the life cycle of *Neurospora*, be certain to review it carefully. Be certain to consider terms such as *prototroph* and *auxotroph*. *Neurospora* is a haploid organism that can be grown on minimal medium (carbon source such as glucose or sucrose, various salts, and biotin), thereby providing an opportunity to define, to some extent, the molecular environments of life. Mutational upset interferes with normal metabolic processes and provides a window to examine such processes and even "cure" them by additives to the minimal medium. Mating types occur that allow one to make crosses, follow segregation patterns, and map genes. While prototrophs are able to grow on minimal medium, auxotrophs (nutritionally mutant strains) are unable to do so unless provided supplements: **A**, **B**, or **C** in this problem. Growth (+) occurs when a prototroph is placed on complete, minimal, or minimal plus supplement(s) medium. For an auxotroph to grow, it must be placed on complete medium or medium with the proper supplement. Any supplement will not suffice. Only supplements that occur after the metabolic block will allow growth of an auxotroph. Study the example below:

Consider the following simple metabolic pathway:

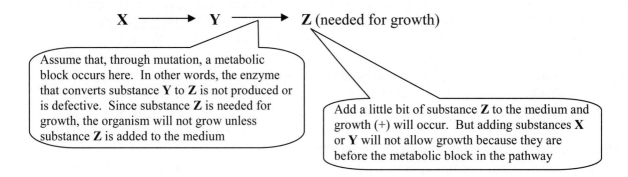

Two important conclusions can be reached from the relationships spelled out above. First, components of a metabolic pathway can be ordered in sequence, and second, the positions of the metabolic blocks can be determined. These two conclusions can be reached by applying the following concept: if a substance "cures" an auxotroph, it must be after the metabolic block in the pathway. If curing does not occur, that substance is either unrelated to the pathway, or it occurs before the metabolic block.

One of the biggest problems beginning students have with this type of problem is keeping the strains and additives straight.The strains are cultures of *Neurospora* with various names (*967*, *q44*, etc.) that have either no mutations that cause nutritional dependence or some nutritional mutations that make them auxotrophs. Substances **A**, **B**, and **C** are usually amino acids, vitamins, or other nutritional necessities that serve to "cure" auxotrophic strains. Wild-type strains (prototrophs) can make these substances from the meager materials in minimal medium, but auxotrophs lack components (usually enzymes) needed to make necessary substances.

Sentence 3(a): From the table, since strain *q44* is able to grow in the control area (no supplements), it must be the wild-type strain. With regard to the A, B, C pathway, for strain *q44*, there are no apparent mutations.

Sentence 3(b): Applying the concepts presented above, one should consider the following logic when building the pathway. The additive that "cures" the highest number of strains must be at the end of the pathway (because it bypasses the highest number of metabolic blocks). The table shows that additive B must be the terminal substance. Applying the same rationale, additive A "cures" the next highest number of strains; therefore, it must be second from the end. Substance C "cures" the lowest number of strains, so it must occur earliest in the pathway. The answer to part (b) is therefore the following sequence of additives.

C ⟶ A ⟶ B (needed for growth)

Sentence 3(c): The placement of the mutations defining each strain is simplified by considering that if a mutational block occurs early, most or all of the additives will be after the block and therefore most or all will "cure" that strain. If a mutational block occurs late in the pathway, only the last additive will "cure" that strain. Applying this logic, we see that strain 967 is "cured" by all three additives; therefore, it must occur before C. Consider that there would be some precursor before additive C and the block occurred between some precursor and additive C. Applying the same logic to the other strains, one can place blocks in the following places.

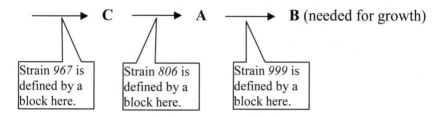

Question 3: Level 2

Three independently assorting genes control the pigmentation biochemical pathway shown below. Genes that produce specific pathway enzymes are noted as *A*, *B*, and *C*. Completely recessive alleles to each gene have been identified as *a*, *b*, and *c*, respectively.

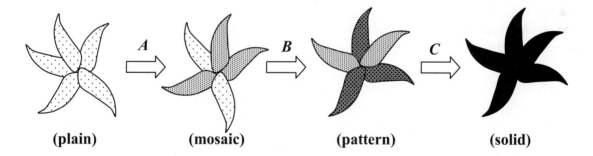

Based on the information provided, give the phenotype and expected frequency (ratio) in the offspring of the following cross: ***AABbCc*** × ***AABbCc***.

Concepts/Processes in Question 3: This question addresses the relationship between **genotypes, phenotypes,** and **epistasis,** in terms of **biochemical pathways**.

Analysis of Question 3:

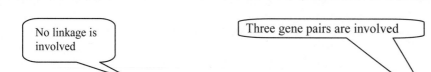

No linkage is involved

Three gene pairs are involved

Level 3. Three independently assorting genes control the pigmentation biochemical pathway shown below.[1] Genes that produce specific pathway enzymes are noted as **A**, **B**, and **C**.[2] Completely recessive alleles to each gene have been identified as **a**, **b**, and **c,** respectively.[3]

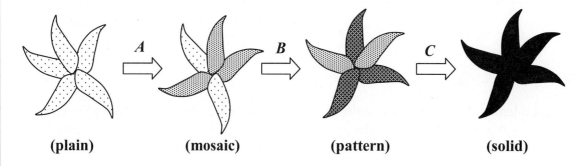

| (plain) | (mosaic) | (pattern) | (solid) |

Based on the information provided, give the phenotype and expected frequency (ratio) in the offspring of the following cross: **AABbCc × AABbCc**.[4]

Calling for only a few of the possible combinations (notice the **A** locus is homozygous dominant, not heterozygous). Apply the forked-line method if needed, but there is an obvious shortcut

---

Sentences 1 and 2: The first sentence and the diagram indicate a linear biochemical pathway controlled by three independently assorting gene pairs. At this point, one would expect that any mutations in the pathway would block the pathway at specific points.

Sentence 3: Homozygosity for any one of the three recessive alleles should block the pathway at its respective steps. Since this is a linear pathway and all three gene pairs influence the same pathway, one might expect to see **epistasis,** whereby mutations early in the pathway would render later mutations insignificant and undetectable by direct observation.

Sentence 4 and answer: While the cross (*AABbCc* × *AABbCc*) involves three independently segregating loci, only two of the loci are heterozygous. Therefore, the answer can be easily obtained by applying the forked-line method. However, because each parent is a double heterozygote (*AABbCc* × *AABbCc*) for the **B** and **C** loci, the problem resolves into a simple 9:3:3:1 dihybrid ratio with epistasis.

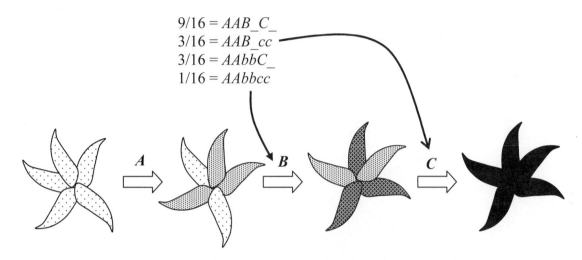

$$9/16 = AAB\_C\_$$
$$3/16 = AAB\_cc$$
$$3/16 = AAbbC\_$$
$$1/16 = AAbbcc$$

If one now applies the appropriate phenotypes based on the positions of the metabolic blocks, the following answers emerge:

$$9/16 = AAB\_C\_ \implies \text{solid}$$
$$3/16 = AAB\_cc \implies \text{pattern}$$
$$3/16 = AAbbC\_ \implies \text{mosaic}$$
$$1/16 = AAbbcc \implies \text{mosaic}$$

These have the identical phenotype because of **epistasis** and are grouped together for a final ratio of 9:3:4.

The answer is 9/16 are solid, 3/16 are pattern, and 4/16 are mosaic.

The following diagram represents gene expression in a model organism. The arrow indicates the direction of movement (left to right) of the transcriptional protein attached to one of the DNA strands.

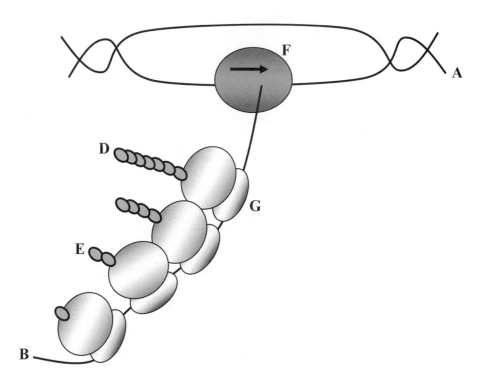

(a) To which end of the DNA (5' or 3') is letter **A** closest?

(b) What is the name of the nucleic acid closest to letter **B**?

(c) To which end (5' or 3') is letter **B** closest?

(d) Assume that letter **D** is closest to the amino acid f-methionine. Is a f-methionine most likely closest to letter **E** also?

(e) Is this diagram depicting processes in eukaryotes or prokaryotes?

(f) What is name of the transcriptional protein closest to letter **F**?

(g) What structure is closest to letter **G**?

Concepts/Processes in Question 4: This question addresses **transcription** and **translation** in a **prokaryote**.

Analysis of Question 4:

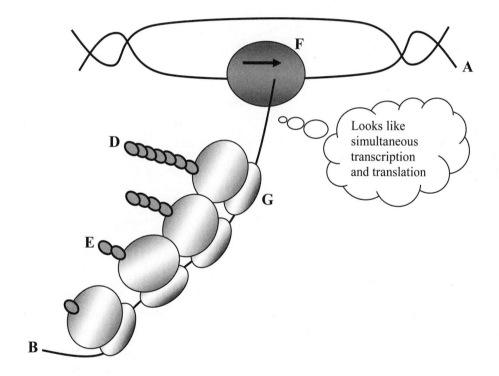

> We typically think of transcription and translation as fundamental components of protein synthesis

> There is no indication of whether the model organism is prokaryotic or eukaryotic

Level 3. The following diagram represents gene expression in a model organism.[1] The arrow indicates the direction of movement (left to right) of the transcriptional protein attached to one of the DNA strands.[2]

> Looks like simultaneous transcription and translation

(a) To which end of the DNA (5' or 3') is letter **A** closest?[3]

(b) What is the name of the nucleic acid closest to letter **B**?[4]

(c) To which end (5' or 3') is letter **B** closest?[5]

(d) Assume that letter **D** is closest to the amino acid f-methionine.[6] Is a f-methionine most likely closest to letter **E** also?[7]

(e) Is this diagram depicting processes in eukaryotes or prokaryotes?[8]

(f) What is name of the transcriptional protein closest to letter **F**?[9]

(g) What structure is closest to letter **G**?[10]

Sentence 1: Gene expression is composed of two major steps: transcription and translation. Each step should come to mind when the process of gene expression arises.

Sentence 2: Since the transcriptional protein is located on a strand of DNA and appears to be producing an mRNA, as evidenced by a string of bound ribosomes, this protein is likely to be a RNA polymerase. Both transcription and translation are occurring simultaneously, indicating that the diagram is representative of gene expression in a prokaryote.

Sentence 3 and answer (a): All nucleic acid synthesis copies the template from the 3' to 5' direction and builds products from the 5' to 3' direction. That is, each new nucleotide is added at the 3' end of a growing strand, as indicated in the diagram below:

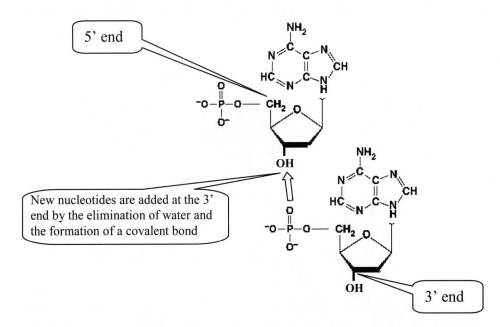

Since the polymerase is moving from left to right according to the arrow, it must be copying (making an RNA strand based on complementarity) from the 3' to the 5' direction. Therefore, letter **A** must be nearest to the 5' end of the template DNA strand. There is another way to arrive at the correct answer. The beginning of the transcript (nearest letter **B**) must be the 5' end since it was the first to be made, given the 5' to 3' nature of nucleic acid synthesis. If you hold the 5' end of the transcript away from the direction of the arrow in the polymerase, it must be complementary to the 3' end of the DNA strand, as pictured below:

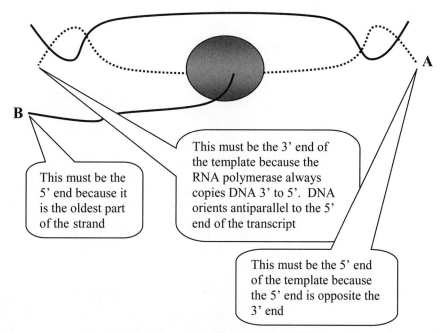

Sentence 4 and answer (b): Notice that the strand nearest letter **B** has what appear to be ribosomes attached with growing polypeptide chains. It must therefore be an mRNA.

Sentence 5 and answer (c): As discussed earlier, all synthesis of nucleic acids occurs in the 5' to 3' direction. Therefore, the oldest portion of a strand is the 5' end and the newest is the 3' end. Since the RNA polymerase is adding new nucleotides at the 3' end, letter **B** must be nearest to the 5' end.

Sentence 6: Methionine, or more correctly, a derivative of methionine (*N*-formylmethionine), is the first amino acid coded for in prokaryotes (methionine in eukaryotes).

Sentence 7 and answer (d): The same mRNA is being translated by each ribosome, the only difference being how far along they are in the process. Since the same mRNA is being translated, all the amino acid sequences should be identical and start with the same amino acid.

Sentence 8 and answer (e): In eukaryotes, transcription occurs in the nucleus and translation occurs in the cytoplasm. However, in prokaryotes, transcription and transcription can occur simultaneously, as pictured in the diagram. This is a sketch of simultaneous transcription and translation in prokaryotes.

Sentence 9 and answer (f): As mentioned earlier, it looks as if this diagram depicts simultaneous transcription and translation. The enzyme that is bound to the DNA that appears to be making an mRNA must be RNA polymerase.

Sentence 10 and answer (g). Ribosomes attach to the mRNA during the process of translation, which is depicted in the diagram. Specifically, nearest letter **G** is the small subunit of the ribosome.

To the right is a table representing the codon assignments for the 20 amino acids as well as the three stop codons.

(a) Select an amino acid that shows that the code is degenerate or that synonyms exist.

(b) Select an amino acid that serves as a chain initiator.

(c) Provide a triplet that serves as a signal to stop translation of a given mRNA.

(d) Of the three bases in a synonymous triplet, which is most variable, first, second, or third?

(e) Select an amino acid that has more than four synonymous codons.

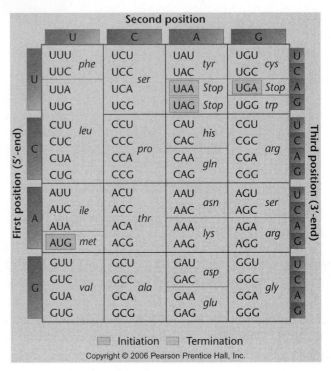

Concepts/Processes in Question 5: The general architecture of the genetic code is addressed in this problem: **degeneracy**, **synonyms, punctuation** (**initiation** and **termination**), and **structure**.

Analysis of Question 5:

> Codons are three-base sequences that specify various amino acids as well as initiate and terminate a coding sequence

Level 1. To the right is a table representing the codon assignments for the 20 amino acids as well as the three stop codons.[1]

(a) Select an amino acid that shows that the code is degenerate or that synonyms exist.[2]

(b) Select an amino acid that serves as a chain initiator.[3]

(c) Provide a triplet that serves as a signal to stop translation in a given mRNA.[4]

(d) Of the three bases in a synonymous triplet, which is most variable, first, second, or third?[5]

(e) Select an amino acid that has more than four synonymous codons.[6]

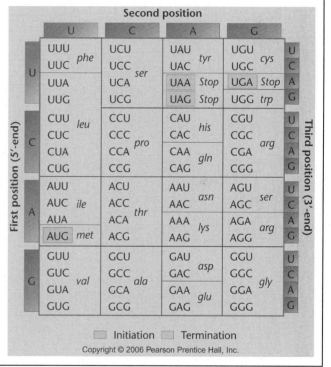

Second position

	U	C	A	G	
U	UUU UUC *phe* UUA UUG	UCU UCC UCA UCG *ser*	UAU UAC *tyr* UAA *Stop* UAG *Stop*	UGU UGC *cys* UGA *Stop* UGG *trp*	U C A G
C	CUU CUC CUA CUG *leu*	CCU CCC CCA CCG *pro*	CAU CAC *his* CAA CAG *gln*	CGU CGC CGA CGG *arg*	U C A G
A	AUU AUC AUA *ile* AUG *met*	ACU ACC ACA ACG *thr*	AAU AAC *asn* AAA AAG *lys*	AGU AGC *ser* AGA AGG *arg*	U C A G
G	GUU GUC GUA GUG *val*	GCU GCC GCA GCG *ala*	GAU GAC *asp* GAA GAG *glu*	GGU GGC GGA GGG *gly*	U C A G

First position (5'-end) — Third position (3'-end)

☐ Initiation ☐ Termination

Copyright © 2006 Pearson Prentice Hall, Inc.

Sentence 1: The table is presented in a fairly standard format with the first base on the left, the second base at the top, and the third base on the right. The first base for each codon starts the 5' end of the coding sequence on an mRNA.

Sentence 2 and answer (a): Notice that in most cases, there is more than one codon for a given amino acid. In other words, the code has synonyms, and is therefore called degenerate. Any amino acid other than tryptophan (trp) and methionine (met) would qualify as a correct answer.

Sentence 3 and answer (b): One amino acid, methionine (met), with the codon AUG, is the chain initiator in both prokaryotes and eukaryotes. AUG will occur at the 5' end of the coding sequence of an mRNA.

Sentence 4 and answer (c): There are three base sequences that do not code for an amino acid: UAA, UGA, and UAG. These are called termination or stop codons. Thus, 61 codons are used for amino acids, while three are used in termination of a coding sequence.

Sentences 5 and 6 and answers (d) and (e): Of the three bases in synonymous codons, the third base is the most variable. In some cases the first base varies as well, as is the case with serine, arginine, and leucine, each encoded by six different codons.

Question 6: Level 2

Provide a possible sequence of nucleotides in the *DNA template strand* for an mRNA that codes for the polypeptide sequence N-His-Arg-Tyr-C.

A. 5'-CAUCGUUAU-3'
B. 3'- CAUCGUUAU -5'
C. 5'- GTAGCAATA -3'
D. 5'- CATCGTTAT-3'
E. 5' – ATAACGATG – 3'

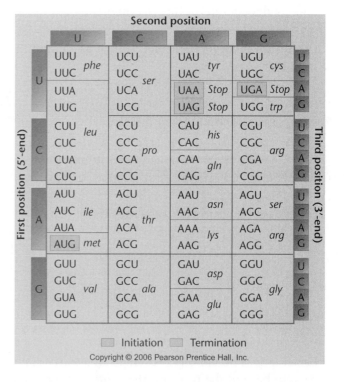

Concepts/Processes in Question 6: There are several main concepts in this question. First, it is necessary to understand that each amino acid in the chain will have at least one **codon** in the table. One reads the codons from the **5' to the 3' end** starting with the **N (amino) terminus** of the polypeptide chain. Second, one must deal with base **complementarity** to determine the DNA sequence from an RNA strand, keeping in mind the **antiparallel** nature of nucleic acids.

Analysis of Question 6:

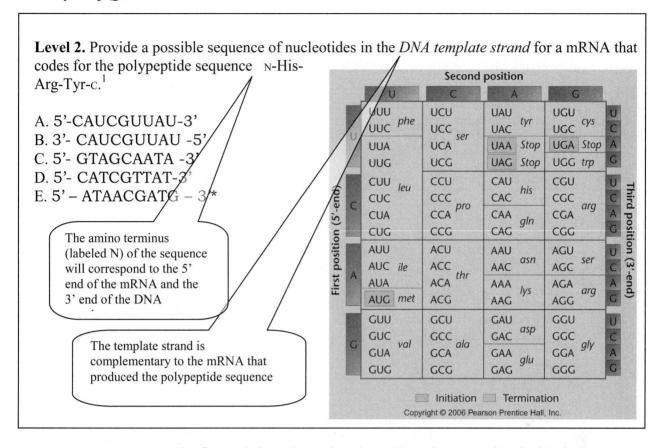

Level 2. Provide a possible sequence of nucleotides in the *DNA template strand* for a mRNA that codes for the polypeptide sequence N-His-Arg-Tyr-c.[1]

A. 5'-CAUCGUUAU-3'
B. 3'- CAUCGUUAU -5'
C. 5'- GTAGCAATA -3'
D. 5'- CATCGTTAT-3'
E. 5' – ATAACGATG – 3'*

The amino terminus (labeled N) of the sequence will correspond to the 5' end of the mRNA and the 3' end of the DNA

The template strand is complementary to the mRNA that produced the polypeptide sequence

Initiation   Termination

Sentence 1 and answer: The first task is to determine the RNA codons associated with the polypeptide chain, keeping in mind that the N terminus of the chain corresponds to the 5' end of the mRNA. Below are the possible codons for the sequence:

   His CA(U,C)   *Arg* CG(U,C,A,G), AG(A,G)   *Tyr* UA(U,C)

The mRNA that would specify such a polypeptide could be simplified by the following:

   5' – CA? CG? UA? – 3'
             AG?

The complementary DNA strand (thus the template strand) would have the following general formula: 3' – GT? GC? AT? – 5'
                                                                   TC?

The first two answers can be eliminated immediately because there is a uracil (U) in the sequence and DNA does not normally contain uracil. Of the last three, obeying 5' – 3' polarity requirements, answer E gives the correct sequence.

Dugaiczyk (1979) and Chambon (1981) used chicken (*Gallus domesticus*) ovalbumin RNA in a hybridization experiment with denatured chicken DNA. Electron microscopy revealed a number of loops, as sketched below. Identify with an "X" the true statements below.

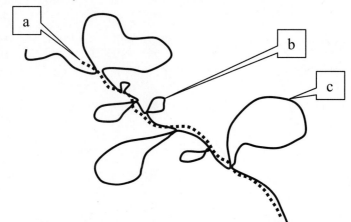

(a) _____ Pointer "a" most likely identifies a primary transcript, before processing.

(b) _____The small loop at letter "b" represents an intron.

(c) _____ The loop at "c" indicates a large exon

(d) _____ The dotted line most likely represents mature mRNA.

(e) _____ The solid line represents DNA.

Concepts/Processes in Question 7: The processes of eukaryotic **mRNA processing** along with **RNA/DNA hybridization** are addressed. **Introns** and **exons** are identifiable by such hybridization.

Analysis of Question 7:

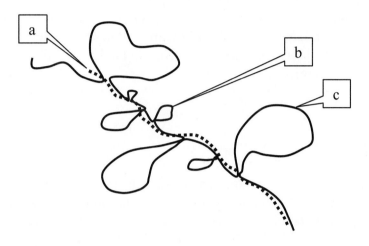

Ovalbumin is an egg protein secreted by the oviducts. The type of RNA is not specified

Level 3. Dugaiczyk (1979) and Chambon (1981) used chicken (*Gallus domesticus*) ovalbumin RNA in a hybridization experiment with denatured chicken DNA.[1] Electron microscopy revealed a number of loops, as sketched below.[2] Identify with an "X" the true statements below.

(a) _____ Pointer "a" most likely identifies a primary transcript, before processing.[3]
(b) _____ The small loop at letter "b" represents an intron.[4]
(c) _____ The loop at "c" indicates a large exon.[5]
(d) _____ The dotted line most likely represents mature mRNA.[6]
(e) _____ The solid line represents DNA.[7]

Sentence 1: An RNA species is being hybridized to denatured DNA. When denatured, the DNA is rendered single stranded, thus exposing the nucleotide bases to complementary bases on the RNA. RNA/DNA hybrids are made to the ovalbumin RNA, most likely mRNA because a particular type of RNA has been identified.

Sentence 2: Looping indicates that certain portions of one strand (the solid line of the loops) are not present in the other strand (the dotted line). At this point, one might consider a processing of a primary transcript, probably an ovalbumin mRNA.

Sentence 3 and answer (a): If the RNA was hybridized before processing, there would be no looping. Therefore, answer (a) is not true.

Sentence 4 and answer (b): Introns are spliced out of a primary transcript in the process of making a eukaryotic mRNA. A loop would be expected in the DNA section that contains an intron. Therefore, (b) is a correct statement.

Sentence 5 and answer (c): Loops represent introns in the DNA, not exons. Therefore, (c) is not correct.

Sentence 6 and answer (d): Since mRNA are products of processing, including the removal of introns, and therefore loops would form in DNA if introns were present in that DNA, it is likely that the dotted line represents exons and answer (d) is correct.

Sentence 7 and answer (e): All the information is consistent with the solid line being DNA and the dotted line being a fully processed mRNA. An ovalbumin mRNA is being hybridized to the gene that makes that RNA. The loops represent the introns in the DNA, while the exons in the DNA are fully hybridized to the mRNA.

Question 8: Level 3

Assume that the partial template strand of wild-type gene pictured below undergoes a series of mutations. For each mutation, using the genetic code, present the new amino acid sequence and state the category of the mutation (nonsense, missense, frameshift, or trinucleotide repeat).

Partial coding strand: 3'- T A C C G G C T A A C A A T A G A T C C T...

(a) 3'- T A C C G G C T A A C A <u>A A A</u> G A T C C T...
(b) 3'- T A C C G G C T A A C A <u>A C A A C A</u> A T A...
(c) 3'- T A C C G|C T A A C A A T A G A T C C T A...

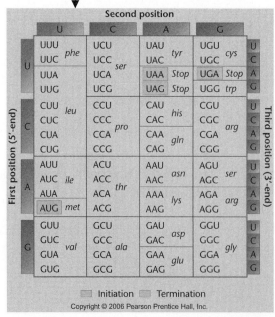

172

Concepts/Processes in Question 8: There are several concepts in this question. First, one must understand that the **template strand of DNA** is involved in the synthesis of RNA in this context. The RNA will be synthesized in the 5' to 3' direction **antiparallel** to the DNA template strand. Second, as changes occur in the coding strand, complementary changes occur in the mRNA, which are then revealed as changes in the amino acid sequence. Third, there are four types of mutations described: **nonsense**, **missense**, **frameshift**, and **trinucleotide repeat**.

Analysis of Question 8:

A mutation is any one or combination of changes in DNA that may or may not influence the phenotype

The template strand is complementary to the mRNA that produces the polypeptide sequence

Level 3. Assume that the partial template strand of wild-type gene pictured below undergoes a series of mutations.[1] For each mutation, using the genetic code, present the new amino acid sequence and state the category of the mutation (nonsense, missense, frameshift, or trinucleotide repeat).[2]

These are common categories, but not all inclusive, of mutations

Partial coding strand: 3'- T A C C G G C T A A C A A T A G A T C C T...[3]

   (a) 3'- T A C C G G C T A A C A <u>A A A</u> G A T C C T...[4]
   (b) 3'- T A C C G G C T A A C A <u>A C A A C A</u> A T A ...[5]
   (c) 3'- T A C C G|C T A A C A A T A G A T C C T A...[6]

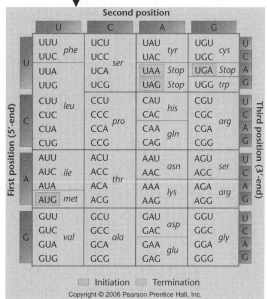

Sentence 1: Since transcription proceeds from the 3' to the 5' end of the strand being copied, it is convenient to write the template strand of the DNA to start from the 3' end. Mutations should consist of various changes in the base sequence of the DNA.

Sentence 2: Because the template DNA strand is provided, it would be easiest to transcribe the mRNA for each mutation, then, using the code table, fill in the appropriate amino acid sequence. A nonsense mutation is one in which a stop codon is brought into the coding sequence, while a missense mutation will call in (substitute) the wrong amino acid. Frameshift mutations shift the reading frame and usually cause multiple amino acid substitutions or termination downstream. Trinucleotide repeats bring in a string of the same amino acid.

Sentence 3: The wild-type DNA template strand, its complementary RNA, and amino acid chain would be as follows:

```
3'- T A C  C G G  C T A  A C A  A T A  G A T  C C T....... DNA template
5'- A U G  G C C  G A U  U G U  U A U  C U A  G G A....... mRNA
     met    ala    asp    cys    tyr    leu    gly      amino acids
```

Sentence 4 and answer (a): Notice that a T > A change (missense) occurs, replacing tyrosine with phenylalanine.

```
3'- T A C  C G G  C T A  A C A  A A A  G A T  C C T....... DNA template
5'- A U G  G C C  G A U  U G U  U U U  C U A  G G A....... mRNA
     met    ala    asp    cys    phe    leu    gly      amino acids
```

Sentence 5 and answer (b): Notice that two additional trinucleotides are present (UCU), thereby leading to a string of three *cys* amino acids.

```
3'- T A C  C G G  C T A  A C A  A C A  A C A  A T A....... DNA template
5'- A U G  G C C  G A U  U G U  U C U  U G U  U A U....... mRNA
     met    ala    asp    cys    cys    cys    tyr      amino acids
```

Sentence 6 and answer (c): Notice that a G is missing at the start of the template DNA, which changes the reading frame downstream. Such a change, alters corresponding amino acids. In addition, notice that a UAG codon (nonsense in this context) that terminated the chain was introduced.

```
3'- T A C  C G C  T A A  C A A  T A G  A T C  C T....... DNA template
5'- A U G  G C G  A U U  G U U  A U C  U A G  G A....... mRNA
     met    ala    ile    val    ile   STOP          amino acids
```

174

Session VIII

Genetic Regulation in Prokaryotes: Who Tells Whom What to Do and When to Do It***

Concepts/Processes	Level(s)	Relevant Question(s)	Page(s)
Inducible/repressible systems	1	1	176
Positive/negative control	2	2	179
***Lac* operon**	2	3	181
***Trp* operon, structure**	2	4	183
***Trp* operon, attenuation**	2, 3	4, 5	183, 185
***Lac* operon genotypes**	2	6	187
***Lac* operon mutations**	2, 3	6, 7	187, 190
***Lac* operon, *cis/trans*, dominance**	4	8	194
Catabolite Repression	2	9	198
Sample Problem	3	10	200

*While an understanding of genetic regulation in eukaryotes is critically important, such processes are usually taught in a more descriptive than analytical fashion at the introductory level, and are therefore not discussed in this handbook. In addition, when such problems are presented to students, they tend to follow some of the same logic (but through different mechanisms) associated with regulation in prokaryotes.

**There are numerous and varied mechanisms of genetic regulation in prokaryotes. The attempt here is to concentrate on developing an in-depth understanding of the fundamentals of analytical approaches to genetic regulation in two classic systems, lactose and tryptophan utilization. Students will most often be expected to master one or both of these systems and develop a basic understanding of how such models are developed. Such an understanding can then be applied to other regulatory mechanisms. It is beyond the scope of this handbook to provide analytical approaches to all regulatory systems in prokaryotes. Most notably, problems associated with bacteriophage lambda are omitted.

Two classic examples provided the early framework for our understanding of genetic regulation in bacteria: lactose utilization and tryptophan synthesis. Below is a table in which you are to first provide an example (A) of each type of regulation and then state (*yes* or *no*) whether operon transcription occurs under the conditions specified by conditions B, C, and D.

	Inducible Operon	Repressible Operon
A. Example		
	Operon Transcription	
B. Lactose added to medium		
C. Tryptophan added to medium		
D. Repressor bound to operator		

Concepts/Processes in Question 1: This question addresses **inducible** and **repressible** **processes** in two classic regulatory systems in bacteria: *lac* and *trp*.

A rather thorough understanding of these two examples is necessary for understanding basic concepts of genetic regulation

Analysis of Question 1:

Level 1. Two classic examples provided the early framework for our understanding of genetic regulation in bacteria: lactose utilization and tryptophan synthesis.[1] Below is a table in which you are to first provide an example (A) of each type of regulation and then state (*yes* or *no*) whether operon transcription occurs under the conditions specified by conditions B, C, and D.[2]

An operon is a cluster of regulatory and structural genes whose expression is under coordinate control

	Inducible Operon	Repressible Operon
A. Example		
	Operon Transcription	
B. Lactose added to medium		
C. Tryptophan added to medium		
D. Repressor bound to operator		

Sentence 1: There are two classic examples that typify inducible and repressible regulatory systems in bacteria. Lactose, a disaccharide made of glucose and galactose, can be metabolized if the lactose operon transcribes its structural genes. The *trp* operon is regulated by levels of tryptophan, an amino acid. Knowledge of both systems provided the conceptual infrastructure for understanding regulation in bacteria and to a great extent viruses and eukaryotes.

Sentence 2: First, let's define the terms inducible and repressible.

An *inducible* operon is one that is turned on, is transcribed, under the influence of a chemical substance in the medium. In the case of the *lac* operon, lactose (or allolactose) alters the conformation of the repressor (product of the *lacI*$^+$ gene, not part of the operon *per se*) so that it can not bind to the operator (*lacO*$^+$). In the absence of repressor binding, the structural genes (β-galactosidase, permease, and transacetylase) are transcribed. Therefore, in the presence of lactose, the operon is *induced*.

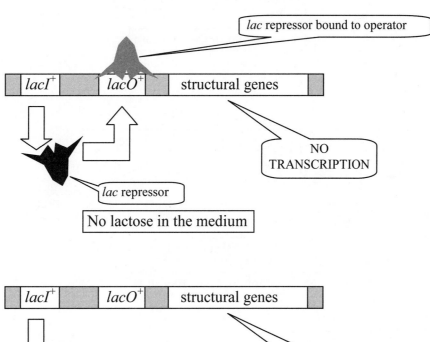

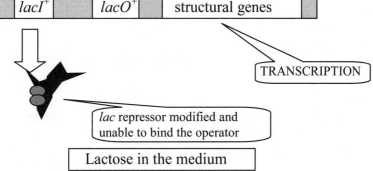

A *repressible* operon is one in which a chemical in the medium winds up shutting off (repressing) transcription of the structural genes of an operon. In the case of the *trp* operon, the repressor produced by the (*trpR*) gene is *normally inactive*. In the presence of tryptophan, its conformation is altered and it becomes capable of binding with the operator (*trpO*). Such binding shuts off transcription; thus the system is repressed by a chemical in the medium.

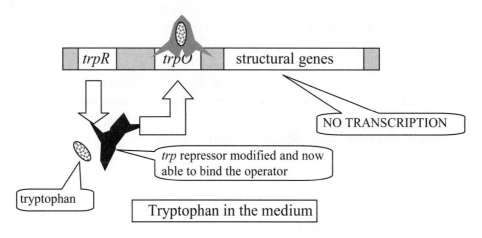

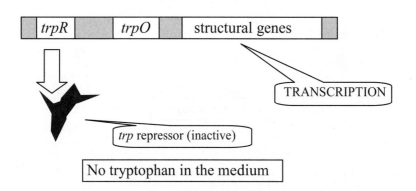

Answers to Question 1:

	Inducible Operon	Repressible Operon
A. Example	*lac*	*trp*
	Operon Transcription	
B. Lactose added to medium	*yes*	*yes*
C. Tryptophan added to medium	*no*	*no*
D. Repressor bound to operator	*no*	*no*

Question 2 :Level 2

Two classic examples provided the early framework for our understanding of genetic regulation in bacteria: lactose utilization (*lac*) and tryptophan synthesis (*trp*). In addition to describing them as inducible and repressible, they also illustrate more general forms of regulation. Negative control occurs when a repressor molecule binds to an operon and inhibits transcription. Positive control occurs when an activator binds to a section of DNA and facilitates transcription. Indicate which of the two forms of genetic control (*negative* and/or *positive*) is(are) associated with these two operons.

lac operon: _____

trp operon: _____

Concepts/Processes in Question 2: This question addresses the two major categories of interaction of an operon with a regulatory protein: **positive** and **negative** control.

Analysis of Question 2:

Negative and positive control (next sentence) issues are at the heart of genetic regulation

Level 2. Two classic examples provided the early framework for our understanding of genetic regulation in bacteria: lactose utilization (*lac*) and tryptophan synthesis (*trp*).[1] In addition to describing them as inducible and repressible, they also illustrate more general forms of regulation.[2] Negative control occurs when a repressor molecule binds to an operon and inhibits transcription.[3] Positive control occurs when an activator binds to a section of DNA and facilitates transcription.[4] Indicate which of the two forms of genetic control (*negative* and/or *positive*) is(are) associated with these two operons.[5]

lac operon: _____

trp operon: _____

If transcription is facilitated, it is more likely to occur, assuming other factors are in place

In this context, repressor and activator molecules are proteins that can bind to DNA

Sentence 1: There are two classic examples that typify inducible and repressible regulatory systems in bacteria. Lactose, a disaccharide made of glucose and galactose, can be metabolized if the lactose operon transcribes its structural genes. The *trp* operon is regulated by levels of tryptophan, an amino acid. Knowledge of both systems provided the conceptual infrastructure for understanding regulation in bacteria and to a great extent viruses and eukaryotes.

Sentence 2: In addition to inducible and repressible conditions, in which medium-supplied substances interact with either active or inactive repressors, respectively, there are two general modes of interaction of regulatory proteins with DNA. When such an interaction occurs, does the interacting molecule repress transcription or facilitate transcription?

Sentence 3: Under *negative* control, the regulatory protein represses transcription, as shown for both the *lac* and *trp* operons below:

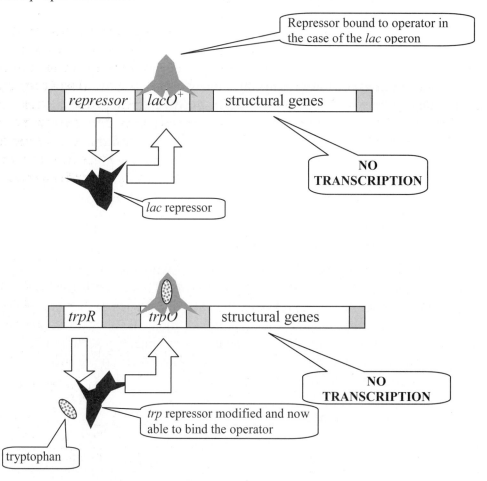

Sentence 4: Under *positive* control, the regulatory protein facilitates transcription, as shown below:

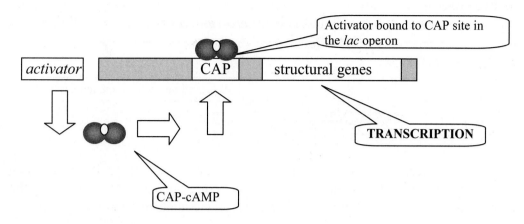

Sentence 5 and answers: Indicate which of the two forms of genetic control (*negative* and/or *positive*) is(are) associated with these two operons.

lac operon:	<u>negative and positive</u>
trp operon:	<u>negative</u>

Question 3: Level 2

The lactose utilization system in *E. coli* is inducible and both positively and negatively regulated. Using the bar below, arrange the following components of *lac* operon and the elements associated with its regulation. Indicate which elements are under coordinate, *cis* induction.

lacZ⁺   *lacO*⁺   *lacI*⁺   *promoter*   *lacY*⁺   *lacZ*⁺   CAPsite   *lac* operon

Concepts/Processes in Question 3: The structure of an operon and its regulatory elements dictates the manner in which regulation can occur: ***cis/trans* control** and **coordinate induction**.

Analysis of Question 3:

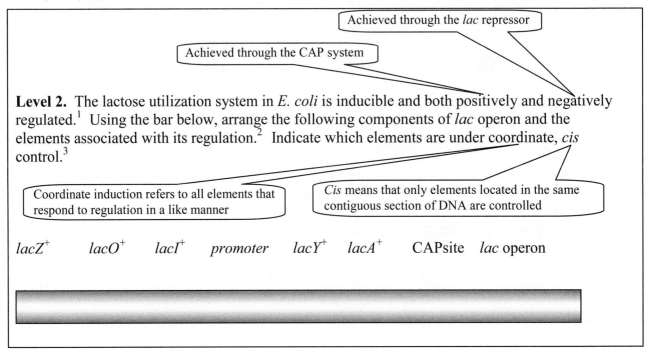

Achieved through the *lac* repressor

Achieved through the CAP system

Level 2. The lactose utilization system in *E. coli* is inducible and both positively and negatively regulated.[1] Using the bar below, arrange the following components of *lac* operon and the elements associated with its regulation.[2] Indicate which elements are under coordinate, *cis* control.[3]

Coordinate induction refers to all elements that respond to regulation in a like manner

Cis means that only elements located in the same contiguous section of DNA are controlled

$lacZ^+$ $lacO^+$ $lacI^+$ *promoter* $lacY^+$ $lacA^+$ CAPsite   *lac* operon

Sentence 1: An *inducible* operon is one that is turned on, is transcribed, under the influence of a chemical substance in the medium. In the case of the *lac* operon, lactose (or allolactose) alters the conformation of the repressor (product of the $lacI^+$ gene) so that it can not bind to the operator ($lacO^+$). In the absence of repressor binding, the structural genes (β-galactosidase, permease, and transacetylase) are transcribed. Therefore, in the presence of lactose, the operon is *induced*. Negative control occurs when a repressor molecule binds to an operon and inhibits transcription. Positive control occurs when an activator binds to a section of DNA and facilitates transcription. See Questions 1 and 2 in this Session for a detailed description of these terms.

Sentence 2 and answer: To arrange components of *lac* operon and the elements associated with its regulation, one should think in terms of each element's function. The operator ($lacO^+$) must sit next to the genes it controls (*cis*-regulation of $lacZ^+$, $lacY^+$, and $lacA^+$), whereas the repressor protein is "diffusable" and therefore functions in *trans*. Below is the overall layout of the *lac* operon and its regulatory elements.

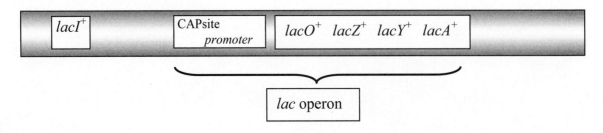

$lacI^+$ CAPsite *promoter* $lacO^+$ $lacZ^+$ $lacY^+$ $lacA^+$

lac operon

Sentence 3 and answer: To say that elements are under coordinate control means that when such elements are induced, they are all induced at the same time and at the same levels. To say that elements behave in *cis*, means that the controlling element must be contiguous (together) in the same DNA strand. If an element is *trans*-controlling, it need not be contiguous with the element(s) under its control. Usually, a *trans*-controlling element is one that can move from place to place and can exert its influence over a distance as, is the case for CAP, and the *lac* and *trp* repressor proteins.

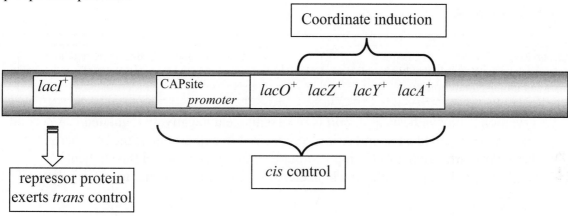

Question 4: Level 2

Tryptophan biosynthesis in *E. coli* is repressible and negatively regulated. A second regulatory mechanism, called attenuation, is also involved in expression of the *trp* operon. Using the bar below, arrange the following components of *trp* operon and the elements associated with its regulation. Indicate which elements are under coordinate, *cis* regulation.

trpR   *trpO*   *promoter*   *leader*   *attenuator*   *trpA*   *trpB*   *trpC*

trpD   *trpE*   *trp* operon

Concepts/Processes in Question 4: The structure and arrangement of genes in the regulatory apparatus of the *trp* operon dictate the conditions under which the structural genes are transcribed. **Cis-repression** is achieved in a typical **negative** manner by binding of an **activated repressor** to the **operator**. **Coordinate induction** occurs because of the **contiguous alignment** of the structural genes, and position of **leader** and **attenuator** sequences allows **attenuation**.

Analysis of Question 4:

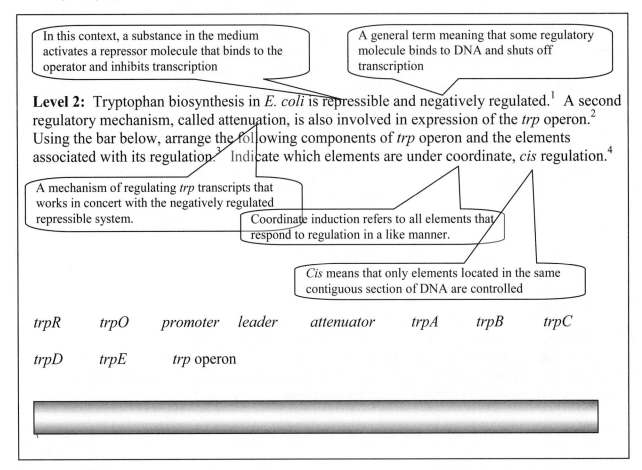

In this context, a substance in the medium activates a repressor molecule that binds to the operator and inhibits transcription

A general term meaning that some regulatory molecule binds to DNA and shuts off transcription

Level 2: Tryptophan biosynthesis in *E. coli* is repressible and negatively regulated.[1] A second regulatory mechanism, called attenuation, is also involved in expression of the *trp* operon.[2] Using the bar below, arrange the following components of *trp* operon and the elements associated with its regulation.[3] Indicate which elements are under coordinate, *cis* regulation.[4]

A mechanism of regulating *trp* transcripts that works in concert with the negatively regulated repressible system.

Coordinate induction refers to all elements that respond to regulation in a like manner.

Cis means that only elements located in the same contiguous section of DNA are controlled

trpR	*trpO*	*promoter*	*leader*	*attenuator*	*trpA*	*trpB*	*trpC*

trpD	*trpE*	*trp* operon

Sentence 1: Tryptophan is an amino acid that can be either taken up from the medium or synthesized within the organism by five structural genes, *trpA* through *trpE*. If tryptophan is in full supply, an inactive repressor is activated that can then bind to the operator and terminate transcription. Because binding of the repressor to the operator leads to a repression of transcription, the *trp* operon is said to be under negative control.

Sentence 2: Attenuation is a second regulatory mechanism in the *trp* operon that works by managing the termination of transcripts of the five *trp* structural genes. (See Question 5 for a more complete description of attenuation.)

Sentence 3: By arranging the elements of *trp* operon, it becomes apparent that the positions occupied by each provides significant underpinnings to the function of the operon.

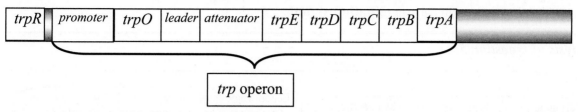

Sentence 4: The elements under coordinate, *cis* regulation are those that operate as a structural and functional unit of contiguous elements.

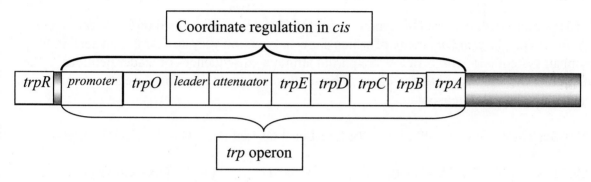

Question 5: Level 3

A number of bacterial biosynthetic operons have been examined in *Escherichia coli* and *Salmonella typhimurium,* many of which show attenuation very similar to that seen in the tryptophan system in *E. coli*. Below are partial amino acid sequences of leader peptides. For each, predict the amino acid that is likely to be synthesized by the operon for each attenuator element. Explain your reasoning.

A. Met-Ser-His-Ile-Val-Arg-Phe-Thr-Gly-Leu-Leu-Leu-Leu-Asn-Ala-Phe-Ile-Val-Arg---

B. Met-Lys-Arg-Ile-Ser-Thr-Thr-Ile-Thr-Thr-Thr-Ile-Thr-Ile-Thr-Thr-Gly-Asn-Gly-Ala---

C. Met-Thr-Arg-Val-Gln-Phe-Lys-His-His-His-His-His-His-His-Pro-Asp---

D. Met-Lys-His-Ile-Pro-Phe-Phe-Phe-Ala-Phe-Phe-Phe-Thr-Phe-Pro---

Answers: **A.**_____   **B.**_____

C._____   **D.**_____

Concepts/Processes in Question 5: Attenuation mediates premature mRNA termination based on the availability of a given amino acid. Under **amino acid deprivation**, genes responsible for the amino acid's synthesis are expressed maximally. Secondary structures of mRNA produce either a **termination** or an **antitermination signal**.

Analysis of Question 5:

> Certain amino acids are synthesized by specific operons that couple negative regulation with attenuation

> Leader regions of operons serve in the mechanism of attenuation by providing regions for mRNA secondary structures to form

Level 3: A number of bacterial biosynthetic operons have been examined in *Escherichia. coli* and *Salmonella typhimurium,* many of which show attenuation very similar to that seen in the tryptophan system in *E. coli*.[1] Below are partial amino acid sequences of leader peptides.[2] For each, predict the amino acid that is likely to be synthesized by the operon for each attenuator element.[3] Explain your reasoning.[4]

A. Met-Ser-His-Ile-Val-Arg-Phe-Thr-Gly-Leu-Leu-Leu-Leu-Asn-Ala-Phe-Ile-Val-Arg---

B. Met-Lys-Arg-Ile-Ser-Thr-Thr-Ile-Thr-Thr-Thr-Ile-Thr-Ile-Thr-Thr-Gly-Asn-Gly-Ala---

C. Met-Thr-Arg-Val-Gln-Phe-Lys-His-His-His-His-His-His-His-Pro-Asp---

D. Met-Lys-His-Ile-Pro-Phe-Phe-Phe-Ala-Phe-Phe-Phe-Thr-Phe-Pro---

Answers: A._____   B. _____

     C._____   D. _____

Sentence 1: A biosynthetic operon is one in which a biologically significant molecule is being made by a coordinately regulated, contiguous group of genes. Attenuation is a process that mediates control over the synthesis of this significant molecule such that if the molecule is in full supply, synthesis is dampened. Attenuation differs from positive/negative control systems in that it involves mRNA transcription termination rather than initiation.

Sentence 2: Attenuation is dependent on a mechanism that assesses internal concentrations of certain biologically significant molecules through the availability of charged tRNAs. If, for example, a Trp-tRNA (charged tryptophanyl-tRNA) is rare because of a short supply of tryptophan, ribosomes translating a leader transcript stall and expose the mRNA to termination because of a particular secondary structure achieved in the leader mRNA sequence.

Sentences 3, and 4 and answers: Since assessing the internal concentrations of a given amino acid is dependent on charged tRNA availability, leader mRNA sequences generally have a strong bias toward codons for the amino acid whose synthesis is to be regulated by attenuation. Therefore; in the coupled transcription/translation process of attenuation, leader peptides that contain a large proportion of a single amino acid are likely to be regulating their own synthesis by attenuation. When examining the partial leader sequences in this question, notice the biases for particular amino acids.

A. Met-Ser-His-Ile-Val-Arg-Phe-Thr-Gly-**Leu-Leu-Leu-Leu**-Asn-Ala-Phe-Ile-Val-Arg---

B. Met-Lys-Arg-Ile-Ser-**Thr-Thr**-Ile-**Thr-Thr-Thr**-Ile-**Thr**-Ile-**Thr-Thr**-Gly-Asn-Gly-Ala---

C. Met-Thr-Arg-Val-Gln-Phe-Lys-**His-His-His-His-His-His-His**-Pro-Asp---

D. Met-Lys-His-Ile-Pro-**Phe-Phe-Phe**-Ala-**Phe-Phe-Phe**-Thr-**Phe**-Pro---

Answers:　　A.　　Leu　　　　B. Thr

　　　　　　　C.　　His　　　　D. Phe

Question 6: Level 2

Much of what is known about genetic regulation in bacteria was discovered through the use of mutations in structural and regulatory genes in the lactose utilization system in *E. coli*. Below is a list of genotypes that played an important role in these discoveries. For each genotype, indicate whether β-galactosidase is produced if lactose is, or is not, provided in the medium. Partial diploids are achieved by additional *lac* genes carried by the F factor. Note: O^C renders the operator insensitive to the repressor and I^- indicates a defective repressor.

Genotype	No Lactose	Lactose	Constitutive
$I^+O^+Z^+$	_____	_____	_____
$I^+O^CZ^+$	_____	_____	_____
$I^-O^+Z^+$	_____	_____	_____
$I^+O^CZ^+/F' I^+O^+Z^+$	_____	_____	_____
$I^+O^+Z^+/F' I^-O^+Z^+$	_____	_____	_____

> **Concepts/Processes in Question 6:** This problem summarizes the relationships between various **genotypes** of the *lac* system and ***lac* operon expression**: **repressed, induced, constitutive,** and **allosteric.**

Analysis of Question 6:

> Lactose inactivates the *lac* repressor, thereby inducing the *lac* operon

> The F factor is a large plasmid that confers fertility to *E. coli*. It can be engineered to carry a variety of genes

Level 2. Much of what is known about genetic regulation in bacteria was discovered through the use of mutations in structural and regulatory genes in the lactose utilization system in *E. coli*.[1] Below is a list of genotypes that played an important role in these discoveries.[2] For each genotype, indicate whether β-galactosidase is produced if lactose is, or is not, provided in the medium.[3] Partial diploids are achieved by additional *lac* genes carried by the F factor.[4] Note: O^C renders the operator insensitive to the repressor and I^- indicates a defective repressor.[5]

> The operon is "on" regardless of lactose in the medium

Genotype	No Lactose	Lactose	Constitutive
$I^+O^+Z^+$	_____	_____	_____
$I^+O^CZ^+$	_____	_____	_____
$I^-O^+Z^+$	_____	_____	_____
$I^+O^CZ^+/F' \ I^+O^+Z^+$	_____	_____	_____
$I^+O^+Z^+/F' \ I^-O^+Z^+$	_____	_____	_____

Sentences 1 and 2: The historical significance of the problem and the question are given.

Sentence 3: The question asks about the production of β-galactosidase, a product of the $lacZ^+$ gene. If lactose is in the medium, then it will interrupt the *lac* repressor and allow β-galactosidase to be made. If there is no lactose in the medium, the *lac* repressor is free to bind to the operator.

Sentence 4: Partial diploids, generated by using an engineered F factor, allow one to test dominance and *cis/trans* relationships in heterozygotes (see Question 8 for development of these issues).

Sentence 5: A variety of mutations in the *lac* operator are known, one being O^C, which renders it insensitive to the repressor. As such, any gene under its control can not be repressed. Of several mutations in the *lacI* gene, I^- fails to make a functional repressor.

Answers:

Genotype	No lactose	Lactose	Constitutive
$I^+O^+Z^+$	no	yes	no

If lactose is in the medium, it will alter the structure of the repressor protein by binding to its allosteric site. The operon will therefore be "on" or induced.

$I^+O^CZ^+$	yes	yes	yes

Because the O^C mutation renders the operator insensitive to the repressor, the operon is always "on" and constitutive production of β-galactosidase occurs.

$I^-O^+Z^+$	yes	yes	yes

Because the I^- mutation renders the repressor ineffective, the operon is always "on" and constitutive production of β-galactosidase occurs.

$I^+O^CZ^+$/F' $I^+O^+Z^+$	yes	yes	yes

With contiguity between O^CZ^+ the condition is set for constitutive production of β-galactosidase, regardless of whether lactose is present in the medium. Since the repressor can not bind to the operator, there is no way to shut down the operon. A repressor-insensitive operator will allow expression of the operon in the presence of a repressor sensitive operator (see Question 8 for further development of this topic).

$I^+O^+Z^+$/F' $I^-O^+Z^+$	no	yes	no

The presence of a defective repressor (I^- in the F factor) does not overcome the influence of a functional repressor (I^+ in the bacterial chromosome) (see Question 8 for further development of the topic of dominant/recessive nature of genes in the *lac* system). Lactose in the medium influences the allosteric site of the repressor and renders it ineffective. Therefore, the *lac* operon is "on" (inducible) when lactose is present in the medium.

For each genotype, indicate the state of the lactose operon if lactose is, or is not, provided in the medium. Partial diploids are achieved by additional *lac* genes carried by the F factor. Note: O^C renders the operator insensitive to the repressor, I^- indicates a defective repressor, and I^s is a mutation that makes the repressor insensitive to lactose..

Genotype/medium	Repressed	Induced	Constitutive
$I^+O^+Z^+$			
No lactose	_____	_____	_____
Lactose	_____	_____	_____
$I^+O^CZ^+$			
No lactose	_____	_____	_____
Lactose	_____	_____	_____
$I^-O^+Z^+$			
No lactose	_____	_____	_____
Lactose	_____	_____	_____
$I^sO^+Z^+$			
No lactose	_____	_____	_____
Lactose	_____	_____	_____
$I^sO^CZ^+$			
No lactose	_____	_____	_____
Lactose	_____	_____	_____
$I^+O^+Z^+/F' \ I^sO^+Z^+$			
No lactose	_____	_____	_____
Lactose	_____	_____	_____
$I^sO^+Z^+/F' \ I^-O^+Z^+$			
No lactose	_____	_____	_____
Lactose	_____	_____	_____

Concepts/Processes in Question 7: This question summarizes the relationships between various **genotypes** of the *lac* system and *lac* **operon expression** under different medium conditions: **repressed**, **induced**, **constitutive**, and **allosteric**.

Analysis of Question 7:

> The F factor is a large plasmid that confers fertility to *E. coli.* It can be engineered to carry a variety of genes

Level 3: For each genotype, indicate the state of the lactose operon if lactose is, or is not, provided in the medium.[1] Partial diploids are achieved by additional *lac* genes carried by the F factor.[2] Note: O^C renders the operator insensitive to the repressor, I^- indicates a defective repressor, and I^s is a mutation that makes the repressor insensitive to lactose.[3]

> The operon is "on" regardless of lactose in the medium

Genotype/medium	Repressed	Induced	Constitutive
$I^+O^+Z^+$			
No lactose	_____	_____	_____
Lactose	_____	_____	_____
$I^+O^CZ^+$			
No lactose	_____	_____	_____
Lactose	_____	_____	_____
$I^-O^+Z^+$			
No lactose	_____	_____	_____
Lactose	_____	_____	_____
$I^sO^+Z^+$			
No lactose	_____	_____	_____
Lactose	_____	_____	_____
$I^sO^CZ^+$			
No lactose	_____	_____	_____
Lactose	_____	_____	_____
$I^+O^+Z^+$/F' $I^sO^+Z^+$			
No lactose	_____	_____	_____
Lactose	_____	_____	_____
$I^sO^+Z^+$/F' $I^-O^+Z^+$			
No lactose	_____	_____	_____
Lactose	_____	_____	_____

Sentence 1: If lactose is not in the medium, the *lac* repressor is free to bind to the operator and shut off transcription (repressed). If lactose is in the medium, then it will interrupt the *lac* repressor and allow β-galactosidase to be made (induced).

Sentence 2: Partial diploids, generated by using an engineered F factor, allow one to test dominance and *cis/trans* relationships in heterozygotes (see Question 8 for development of these issues).

Sentence 3: A variety of mutations in the *lac* operator are known, one being O^C, which renders it insensitive to the repressor. As such, any gene under its control (contiguous) cannot be repressed. Of several mutations in the *lacI* gene, I^- fails to make a functional repressor. I^s is a mutation that makes the repressor insensitive to lactose because the allosteric site on the repressor is altered.

Answers:

Genotype	Repressed	Induced	Constitutive
$I^+O^+Z^+$			
No lactose	yes	no	no
Lactose	no	yes	no

With no lactose in the medium, the repressor is free to bind to the operator and shut off transcription of the *lac* operon. With lactose in the medium, the structure of the repressor protein will be altered and it will not bind to the operator. The operon will therefore be "on" or induced.

Genotype	Repressed	Induced	Constitutive
$I^+O^CZ^+$			
No lactose	no	no	yes
Lactose	no	no	yes

Because the O^C mutation renders the operator insensitive to the repressor, the operon is always "on" and constitutive production of β-galactosidase occurs regardless of the presence or absence of lactose in the medium.

Genotype	Repressed	Induced	Constitutive
$I^-O^+Z^+$			
No lactose	no	no	yes
Lactose	no	no	yes

Because the I^- mutation renders the repressor ineffective, the operon is always "on" and constitutive production of β-galactosidase occurs regardless of the presence or absence of lactose in the medium.

$I^sO^+Z^+$

No lactose	yes	no	no
Lactose	yes	no	no

Because the I^s mutation produces a repressor that is insensitive to lactose, the repressor is active and can interact with the operator. Therefore, regardless of the presence or absence of lactose, the operon is always in the "off" or repressed state.

$I^sO^cZ^+$

No lactose	no	no	yes
Lactose	no	no	yes

O^c will not bind any repressor, including I^s. The operator is insensitive to the repressor. Therefore, regardless of the presence or absence of lactose, the operon is always in the "on" or constitutive state.

$I^+O^+Z^+/F$' $I^sO^+Z^+$

No lactose	yes	no	no
Lactose	yes	no	no

Since lactose works at a site other than the operator-binding site on the repressor (allosteric), the repressor can be insensitive to the inducer (lactose), and still be able to bind to the operator. The operator O^+ is sensitive to the repressor in this case and capable of interacting with the altered repressor. The question is whether I^s will be dominant or recessive to I^+. While this issue will be developed in some detail in Question 8, at this point we can say that in the presence of products of both I alleles, the presence of a lactose-insensitive repressor will mask the presence of a lactose-sensitive repressor. In other words, the addition alters I^+ and renders it unable to bind O^+. But I^s is not changed by lactose. I^s will still bind to O^+, including O^+ previously occupied by I^+ repressors. So, the *lac* operon will be repressed regardless of the presence or absence of lactose in the medium.

$I^sO^+Z^+/F$' $I^-O^+Z^+$

No lactose	yes	no	no
Lactose	yes	no	no

Since lactose works at a site other than the operator-binding site on the repressor (allosteric), the repressor can be insensitive to the inducer (lactose), and still be able to bind to the operator. The operator O^+ is sensitive to the repressor in this case and capable of interacting with the altered repressor. The question is whether I^s will be dominant or recessive to I^-. While this issue will be developed in some detail in Question 8, at this point we can say that the presence of a defective repressor does not mask the presence of a lactose-insensitive repressor. So the *lac* operon will be repressed regardless of the presence or absence of lactose in the medium.

Question 8: Level 4

Below is a list of genotypes that played an important role in the discovery of regulation of lactose utilization in *E. coli*. **(a)** For each genotype, indicate whether functional β-galactosidase is produced if lactose is, or is not, provided in the medium. Partial diploids are achieved by another *lac* operon carried by the F factor. Note: O^C renders the operator insensitive to the repressor, I^- indicates a defective repressor, I^s is a mutation that makes the repressor insensitive to lactose, and Z^- indicates that a mutant, nonfunctional β-galactosidase is produced. **(b)** In the partial diploid genotypes, indicate which of the contrasting alleles O^C vs. O^+, I^- vs. I^+, and I^s vs. I^+ is dominant. **(c)** In the partial diploid genotypes, indicate those that illustrate the *cis* behavior of O^C and those that illustrate the *trans* behavior of I^+.

Genotype/medium	(a) Functional β-galactosidase	(b) Dominant	(c) *Cis/trans*
$I^+O^+Z^+$			
No lactose	_____		
Lactose	_____		
$I^+O^+Z^-$			
No lactose	_____		
Lactose	_____		
$I^-O^+Z^+$			
No lactose	_____		
Lactose	_____		
$I^+O^CZ^+/F'\ I^+O^+Z^-$			
No lactose	_____	_____	_____
Lactose	_____	_____	_____
$I^+O^+Z^+/F'\ I^+O^CZ^-$			
No lactose	_____	_____	_____
Lactose	_____	_____	_____
$I^-O^+Z^+/F'\ I^+O^+Z^-$			
No lactose	_____	_____	_____
Lactose	_____	_____	_____
$I^sO^+Z^+/F'\ I^+O^+Z^+$			
No lactose	_____	_____	_____
Lactose	_____	_____	_____

Concepts/Processes in Question 8: The concepts of **dominance** and *cis/trans* **arrangements** of regulatory genes (O^C vs. O^+, I^- vs. I^+, and I^s vs. I^+) are presented by examining the phenotypes (β-galactosidase production) among various **haploid** and **partial diploid** strains.

Analysis of Question 8:

> Nonfunctional β-galactosidase will be produced by the mutant allele Z^-

Level 4. Below is a list of genotypes that played an important role in the discovery of regulation of lactose utilization in *E. coli*.[1] **(a)** For each genotype, indicate whether functional β-galactosidase is produced if lactose is, or is not, provided in the medium.[2] Partial diploids are achieved by another *lac* operon carried by the F factor.[3] Note: O^C renders the operator insensitive to the repressor, I^- indicates that a defective repressor, I^s is a mutation that makes the repressor insensitive to lactose, and Z^- indicates that a mutant, nonfunctional β-galactosidase is produced.[4] **(b)** In the partial diploid genotypes, indicate which of the contrasting alleles O^C vs. O^+, I^- vs. I^+, and I^s vs. I^+ is dominant.[5] **(c)** In the partial diploid genotypes, indicate those that illustrate the *cis* behavior of O^C and those that illustrate the *trans* behavior of I^+.[6]

> Dominance and recessiveness applies to regulatory genes and operators, as well as structural genes.

> Can the regulatory protein "function at a distance"? Is it contiguous with the element under its control?

Sentence 1: Both classes of genes, regulatory and structural, will be presented in a variety of haploid and partial diploid combinations.

Sentence 2: The question asks about the production of functional β-galactosidase, a product of the *lacZ*$^+$ gene under two medium conditions. If lactose is not in the medium, the *lac* repressor is free to bind to the operator and shut off transcription (repressed). If lactose is in the medium, then it will interrupt the *lac* repressor and allow β-galactosidase to be made (induced). There is the implication that a "nonfunctional" form of the enzyme can be formed. In Sentence 4 is a description of such a case, where a nonfunctional enzyme is formed by a mutation in the *Z* gene.

Sentence 3: Partial diploids, generated by using an engineered F factor, allow one to test dominance and *cis/trans* relationships in heterozygotes.

Sentence 4: A variety of mutations in the *lac* operator are known, one being O^C which renders it insensitive to the repressor. As such, any gene under its control (contiguous) can not be repressed. Of several mutations in the *lacI* gene, I^- fails to make a functional repressor. I^s is a mutation that makes the repressor insensitive to lactose because the allosteric site on the repressor is altered. The Z^- mutation yields a nonfunctional β-galactosidase.

Sentence 5: A determination of dominance is possible when a heterozygous state is present in a partial diploid. The phenotype (β-galactosidase production) can be examined to see which allele prevails in the heterozygous state.

Sentence 6: *Cis* regulatory genes can only influence other genes to which they are connected. That is, if a gene does not produce a diffusible product, its influence can not spread to unconnected DNA sequences. Genes that work in *trans* can influence other genes at a distance. We will see that the operator (*lacO*) operates in *cis*, while the repressor (*lacI*) works in *trans*.

Genotype/medium	(a) Functional β-galactosidase	(b) Dominant	(c) *Cis/trans*

$I^+O^+Z^+$

No lactose	no		
Lactose	yes		

With no lactose in the medium, the repressor is free to bind to the operator and shut off transcription of the *lac* operon. With lactose in the medium, the structure of the repressor protein will be altered and it will not bind to the operator. The operon will therefore be "on" or induced in the presence of lactose.

$I^+O^+Z^-$

No lactose	no		
Lactose	no		

Since there is a mutation in the Z^+ allele to produce the Z^-, nonfunctional enzyme is made regardless of the presence or absence of lactose.

$I^-O^+Z^+$

No lactose	yes		
Lactose	yes		

Because the I^- mutation renders the repressor ineffective, the operon is always "on" and constitutive production of β-galactosidase occurs regardless of the presence or absence of lactose.

$I^+O^CZ^+/F' \; I^+O^+Z^-$

No lactose	yes	O^C is dominant	O^C functions in
Lactose	yes	to O^+	*cis*

Because of the contiguous arrangement of O^CZ^+ there is constitutive production of a functional β-galactosidase. The constitutive phenotype is expressed regardless of the presence of O^+; therefore, O^C is dominant to O^+. Comparing this result to the next one, indicates that O^C works in *cis*; it must be contiguous with genes under its control. Notice that while the genotypes are the same in this partial diploid and the next (only the position of Z^- switched), the phenotype is altered. Therefore, the position of O^C relative to Z determines its function. O^C must function in *cis*.

$I^+O^+Z^+/F' \; I^+O^CZ^-$

No lactose	no		O^C functions in
Lactose	yes		*cis*

Because of the contiguous arrangement of O^CZ^- there is constitutive production of a <u>nonfunctional</u> β-galactosidase; however, a functional β-galactosidase is formed only when lactose interrupts the repressor protein and transcription begins from Z^+. No determination can be made as to the dominance of O^C and O^+ from this partial diploid alone. Comparing this result to the previous one indicates that O^C works in *cis*; it must be contiguous with genes under its control. Notice that while the genotypes are the same in this partial diploid and the one above (only the position of Z^- switched), the phenotype is altered. Therefore, the position of O^C relative to Z determines its function. O^C must function in *cis*.

$I^-O^+Z^+/F' \; I^+O^+Z^-$

No lactose	no	I^+ is dominant	I^+ functions in
Lactose	yes	to I^-	*trans*

Notice that even though I^- is present, the phenotype is influenced only by I^+ thereby indicating that I^+ is dominant to I^-. The only functional repressor is located in the F factor, yet, the only functional β-galactosidase allele is located in the bacterial chromosome. Since repression can occur and functional β-galactosidase is made only when lactose is in the medium, the I^+ allele must work in *trans*.

$I^S O^+ Z^- / F' I^+ O^+ Z^+$

No lactose	no	I^S is dominant	I^S functions in
Lactose	no	to I^+	*trans*

Since lactose works at a site other than the operator-binding site on the repressor (allosteric), the repressor can be insensitive to the inducer (lactose) and still be able to bind to the operator. The operator O^+ is sensitive to the repressor in this case and capable of interacting with the altered repressor. The question is whether I^S will be dominant or recessive to I^-. Even though both repressors, one sensitive to lactose and the other not, are present, a lactose-insensitive repressor can bind to both operators. Since such repressors are not sensitive to lactose, they can continue to bind the operators even in the presence of lactose-sensitive repressors. Therefore, the *lac* operon will be repressed regardless of the presence or absence of lactose in the medium and I^S will behave as a dominant allele to I^-.

The only source for the lactose-insensitive repressor is located in the bacterial chromosome, yet the only functional β-galactosidase allele is located in the F factor. Since lactose-insensitive repression can occur and no functional β-galactosidase is made, the I^S allele must work in *trans*.

Question 9: Level 2

A catabolite-activating protein (CAP) exerts positive control over the *lac* operon. Indicate the level of activity of the *lac* operon under the medium conditions listed below:

(a) No lactose present, no glucose present

(b) Lactose present, no glucose present

(c) No lactose present, glucose present

(d) Lactose present, glucose present

> **Concepts/Processes in Question 9:** The interactions of the *lac* **operon** with the *lacI* and **CAP** (**catabolite repression**) regulatory systems are illustrated.

Analysis of Question 9:

> CAP is activated by cAMP when glucose is not present

> CAP is activated by cAMP and should therefore facilitate transcription of the *lac* operon.

Level 2. A catabolite-activating protein (CAP) exerts positive control over the *lac* operon.[1] Indicate the level of activity of the *lac* operon under the medium conditions listed below:[2]

  (a) No lactose present, no glucose present
  (b) Lactose present, no glucose present
  (c) No lactose present, glucose present
  (d) Lactose present, glucose present

Sentence 1: When CAP is activated by cAMP (CAP-cAMP), it binds to the CAP site upstream from the *lac* operon. In doing so, it facilitates transcription of the *lac* operon.

Sentence 2 and answers: Recall that negative regulation of the *lactose* operon occurs by the *lac* repressor and positive control is exerted by CAP-cAMP. Lactose inactivates the *lac* repressor and glucose inhibits adenyl cyclase, thereby reducing, through a lowering of cAMP levels, the positive transcriptional action of CAP-cAMP on the *lac* operon.

(a) With no lactose and no glucose in the medium, the operon will be off because the *lac* repressor is bound to the operator, and although CAP-cAMP is bound to the CAP site, it can not override the influence of the repressor bound to the operator.

(b) With lactose in the medium, the *lac* repressor is inactivated and the operon can be transcribed. With no glucose in the medium, the CAP-cAMP is bound to the CAP site, thus enhancing transcription. Transcription of the *lac* operon will occur at a high level.

(c) With no lactose in the medium, the *lac* repressor will be bound to the operator, and because glucose inhibits adenyl cyclase, there is no activated CAP (CAP-cAMP) to interact with its binding site. The operon will therefore be "off" is the sense of functioning at relatively low, basal, levels.

(d) With lactose in the medium, the *lac* repressor is inactivated and not functional. However, since glucose is present in the medium, adenyl cyclase will be inhibited and no CAP-cAMP will be formed. The operon will therefore be "off."

Question 10: Level 3

Assume that in a newly discovered bacterial species you discover a cluster of three genes (*A*, *B*, and *C*) that account for the enzymatic production of a cellulose-like carbohydrate (clc) as a component of its cell wall. This cluster of genes appears to be under coordinate control because a deletion in a distant gene (*R*) results in loss of synthesis of all three genes. When clc is in full supply, the three enzymes are not synthesized. When mutations occur (P^-) in a region upstream to gene *A*, no synthesis of the three enzymes occurs, even in the absence of clc.

   (a) Do the three genes (*A*, *B*, and *C*) behave as if they were part of an operon?

   (b) What type of control (*positive* or *negative*) seems likely to control the production of the three enzymes?

   (c) Sketch and label a model that indicates the spatial and functional relationships among all the genetic components described.

Concepts/Processes in Question 10: From these data, a **model** is to be constructed that accounts for the **spatial and functional relationships** that occur in a **typical operon** and **regulatory elements**.

Analysis of Question 10:

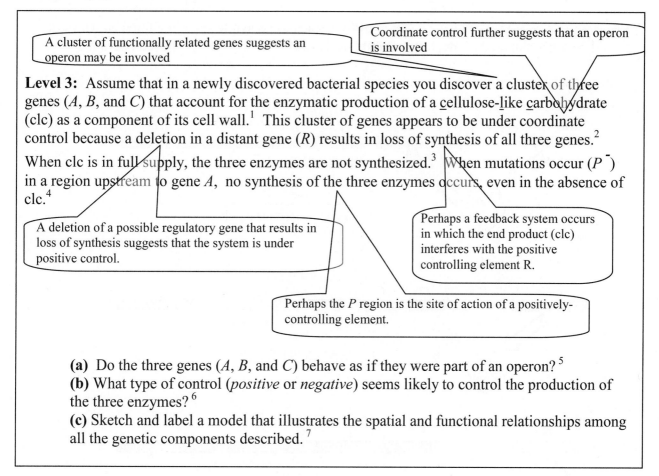

A cluster of functionally related genes suggests an operon may be involved

Coordinate control further suggests that an operon is involved

Level 3: Assume that in a newly discovered bacterial species you discover a cluster of three genes (*A*, *B*, and *C*) that account for the enzymatic production of a cellulose-like carbohydrate (clc) as a component of its cell wall.[1] This cluster of genes appears to be under coordinate control because a deletion in a distant gene (*R*) results in loss of synthesis of all three genes.[2]

When clc is in full supply, the three enzymes are not synthesized.[3] When mutations occur (P^-) in a region upstream to gene *A*, no synthesis of the three enzymes occurs, even in the absence of clc.[4]

A deletion of a possible regulatory gene that results in loss of synthesis suggests that the system is under positive control.

Perhaps a feedback system occurs in which the end product (clc) interferes with the positive controlling element R.

Perhaps the *P* region is the site of action of a positively-controlling element.

(a) Do the three genes (*A*, *B*, and *C*) behave as if they were part of an operon?[5]

(b) What type of control (*positive* or *negative*) seems likely to control the production of the three enzymes?[6]

(c) Sketch and label a model that illustrates the spatial and functional relationships among all the genetic components described.[7]

Sentence 1: The cluster of genes (*A*, *B*, and *C*) accounts for the synthesis of clc, assumed to be a necessary component of the cell wall. This is an anabolic, biosynthesis system much like many involved in amino acid synthesis in bacteria. One would expect that when the end product is in full supply, some mechanism down regulates the production of clc.

Sentence 2: Coordinate control of all three genes by a distant gene (*R*) suggests that a product, R, is involved in the regulation of the three genes. In addition, since removing R results in loss of synthesis of *A*, *B*, and *C*, one might consider that R acts as a *trans*-acting, positive controlling element.

Sentence 3: When clc is in full supply, the positive action of R is removed, suggesting that clc might interfere with the action of R.

Sentence 4: Mutations in *P* lead to no synthesis of the three enzymes and that occurs even in the absence of clc. If *P* is the site of action of a positive controlling element (R), then mutations in *P* would interfere with synthesis of *A*, *B*, and *C*.

Sentence 5 and answer (a): Based on the information presented and the logic applied in the above explanations, it would seem reasonable that genes *A, B*, and *C* belong to an operon.

Sentence 6 and answer (b): Since a deletion of/in *R* leads to no synthesis of the three enzymes, it would be logical that its product, R, exhibits positive control over the proposed operon.

Sentence 7 and answer (c):

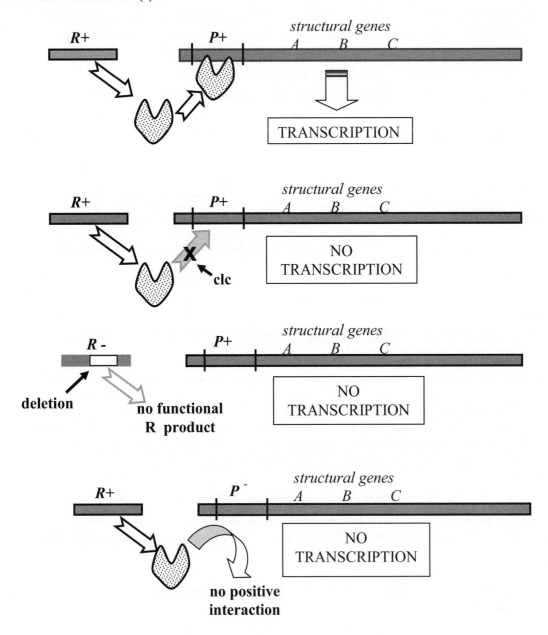

Session IX

Population Genetics: Frequencies of Alleles Through Time and Space

Question 1: Level 1

Assume that you are studying a population of rodents and determine that the frequency of the *A* allele is 0.7 and the frequency of the *a* allele is 0.3. Assume that you sample 1000 rodents in the next generation. Under Hardy-Weinberg conditions, what would you predict as the number of *AA*, *Aa*, and *aa* individuals?

Number of *AA* individuals_____

Number of *Aa* individuals_____

Number of *aa* individuals _____

Concepts/Processes in Question 1: By knowing the frequencies of the *A* (**p**) and the *a* (**q**) alleles, one can compute the **frequencies of homozygotes *AA*, *aa* and heterozygotes** in the next generation under **Hardy-Weinberg conditions**.

Analysis of Question 1:

> Of the two alleles assessed in this population, 7 out of 10 are *A* while 3 out of 10 are *a*

> A population is a group of genetically-related organisms that share a given geographic area and potentially interbreed

Level 1. Assume that you are studying a population of rodents and determine that the frequency of the *A* allele is 0.7 and the frequency of the *a* allele is 0.3.[1] Assume that you sample 1000 rodents in the next generation.[2] Under Hardy-Weinberg conditions, what would you predict as the number of *AA*, *Aa*, and *aa* individuals?[3]

> An "ideal" population that is infinitely large and random mating, without migration, mutation, or selection

Number of *AA* individuals _____

Number of *Aa* individuals _____

Number of *aa* individuals _____

Sentence 1: Allelic frequencies are often estimated using a variety of morphological observations and/or biochemical analyses. If 7 out of 10 alleles are of the *A* type, then the frequency of the *A* allele is said to be 0.7 or $p = 0.7$. Because there are only two alleles described here, the frequency of the other allele *a* must be 0.3 because the total allelic frequencies must equal 1.0. So, $q = 0.3$ and $p + q = 1.0$. In population genetics, one deals with allelic frequencies much as one deals with alleles in Punnett squares, as shown below.

Sentence 2: Generally, in population genetics studies, one is interested in the frequencies of alleles in a comparative sense, by comparing either one population with another or one population with subsequent populations. In this case, the question relates to the numbers of individuals (of 1000) in the *AA*, *Aa*, and *aa* classes in the next generation.

Sentence 3 and answers: The Hardy-Weinberg law states that allelic (*A* and *a*) and genotypic or zygotic (*AA*, *Aa*, and *aa*) frequencies will remain constant in infinitely large, randomly mating populations in which there is no mutation, migration, or selection. While such populations are hypothetical, they represent the starting point for the study of natural populations. In diagram form, one can deal with allelic *frequencies* much like one deals with Mendelian alleles in Punnett squares.

Sperm frequencies from generation 1

$A = 0.7 \ (p)$ $a = 0.3 \ (q)$

These are the combinations for generation 2

Egg frequencies from generation 1

	$A = 0.7$ (p)	$a = 0.3$ (q)
$A = 0.7$ (p)	$AA = 0.7 \times 0.7 = 0.49 \ (p^2)$	$Aa = 0.7 \times 0.3 = 0.21 \ (pq)$
$a = 0.3$ (q)	$Aa = 0.7 \times 0.3 = 0.21 \ (pq)$	$aa = 0.3 \times 0.3 = 0.09 \ (q^2)$

Taking the above values: p^2 = the frequency of AA = 0.49 in generation 2
$2pq$ = the frequency of Aa = 0.21 + 0.21 or 0.42 in generation 2
q^2 = the frequency of aa = 0.09 in generation 2

and multiplying each by 1000 individuals gives the following answers:

Number of AA individuals: 0.49 X 1000 individuals = 490 AA individuals
Number of Aa individuals: 0.42 X 1000 individuals = 420 Aa individuals
Number of aa individuals: 0.09 X 1000 individuals = 90 aa individuals

Finally, when all calculations are complete, it is best to be certain that all components are included and total the expectations:

Theoretical allelic frequencies: $p + q = 1.0$

Actual allelic frequencies: 0.7 + 0.3 = 1.0

Theoretical genotypic (zygotic) frequencies: $p^2 + 2pq + q^2 = 1.0$

Actual genotypic (zygotic) frequencies: 0.49 + 0.42 + 0.09 = 1.0

Actual numbers of individuals: 490 + 420 + 90 = 1000

Assume that you are studying a population of squirrels on the south rim of the Grand Canyon and find that three squirrels out of 300 observed had a unique, solid black color variation. In other mammals, the solid black color variation is caused by a recessive allele, and you assume that to be the case with these squirrels. Under Hardy-Weinberg (HW) assumptions, how many of the 300 squirrels would you assume to be heterozygous?

Concepts/Processes in Question 2: Under HW assumptions, it is possible to estimate **genotypic (zygotic) frequencies** if one knows *p* and/or *q*. The frequency of the recessive allele can be estimated by taking the **square root of the frequency of homozygous recessive individuals**.

Analysis of Question 2:

These values will be used to estimate *q*

Level 2. Assume that you are studying a population of squirrels on the south rim of the Grand Canyon and find that three squirrels out of 300 observed had a unique, solid black, color variation.[1] In other mammals, the solid black color variation is caused by a recessive allele and you assume that to be the case with these squirrels.[2] Under Hardy-Weinberg (HW) assumptions, how many of the 300 squirrels would you assume to be heterozygous?[3]

An "ideal" population that is infinitely large and random mating, without migration, mutation, or selection

Sentences 1 and 2: From information in these two sentences one can compute *q* by taking the square root of the frequency of homozygous recessive individuals.

$$q^2 = 3/300 = 0.01$$

$$q = \sqrt{0.01} = 0.1$$

$$p = 1 - q = 0.9$$

Sentence 3 and answer: Given HW assumptions of an "ideal" population that is infinitely large and random mating, without migration, mutation, or selection, one can estimate the number of heterozygotes by the following procedure.

$$\underline{\text{frequency}} \text{ of heterozygotes} = 2pq = 2 \times 0.9 \times 0.1 = 0.18$$

$$\underline{\text{number}} \text{ of heterozygotes} = 0.18 \times 300 = 54$$

Question 3: Level 2:

The population genetics of sickle cell anemia has been studied all over the world. By using electrophoretic analyses it is possible to determine the genotypes of individuals as *AA*, *AS*, or *SS*. Assume that you are studying a relatively small, isolated South American population and determine the following distribution of genotypes: *AA* = 75; *AS* = 24; *SS* = 1.

(a) Test these data by χ^2 to determine whether these numbers represent a population in HW equilibrium.

(b) Interpret the results of your test in terms of the HW assumptions.

Concepts/Processes in Question 3: This question allows one to **compute *p* and *q* using all genotypic classes**. A χ^2 **test** with one **degree of freedom** will test these data against expectations based on **HW assumptions**.

Analysis of Question 3:

Since all three genotypes are available, a more accurate estimate of p and q will be available

This information may be important when interpreting the distribution data

Level 2. The population genetics of sickle cell anemia has been studied all over the world.[1] By using electrophoretic analyses it is possible to determine the genotypes of individuals as *AA*, *AS*, or *SS*.[2] Assume that you are studying a relatively small, isolated South American population and determine the following distribution of genotypes: *AA* = 75; *AS* = 24; *SS* = 1.[3] **(a)** Test these data by χ^2 to determine whether these numbers represent a population in HW equilibrium.[4] **(b)** Interpret the results of your test in terms of the HW assumptions.[5]

A statistical method for testing "goodness of fit" to a variety of expectations including HW distributions

Sentence 1: Sickle cell anemia is caused by a single amino acid substitution (valine for glutamic acid) in the sixth position of the β chain of hemoglobin. Homozygotes suffer a variety of ailments and sometimes death.

Sentence 2: Electrophoretic separation of hemoglobin can reveal the different charges in the β chains brought about by the substitution of valine for glutamic acid. Identification of such genotypes greatly facilitates studies on the population genetics of sickle cell anemia.

Sentence 3: From the population frequencies, it is possible to compute the allelic frequencies as follows:

$$p = \frac{\text{number of } A \text{ alleles}}{\text{total number of alleles}} = \frac{(2 \times \text{number of } AA \text{ individuals}) + (\text{number of } AS \text{ individuals})}{2 \times \text{total number of individuals}}$$

$$p = \frac{(2 \times 75) + (24)}{2 \times 100} = \frac{174}{200} = 0.87$$

$$q = \frac{\text{number of } S \text{ alleles}}{\text{total number of alleles}} = \frac{(2 \times \text{number of } SS \text{ individuals}) + (\text{number of } AS \text{ individuals})}{2 \times \text{total number of individuals}}$$

$$q = \frac{(2 \times 1) + (24)}{2 \times 100} = \frac{26}{200} = 0.13$$

At this point it is wise to add the values for p and q to be certain that all alleles are accounted for:

$$p + q = 1.0 \qquad\qquad 0.87 + 0.13 = 1.0$$

Sentence 4 and answer (a): From the above values of p and q, the expected numbers of each genotypic class, assuming Hardy-Weinberg conditions, can be computed:

Expected <u>numbers</u> of *AA* genotypes: p^2 X 100 =   0.87 X 0.87 X 100 = 75.69

Expected <u>numbers</u> of *AS* genotypes: $2pq$ X   100 = 2(0.87 X 0.13) X 100 = 22.62

Expected <u>numbers</u> of *SS* genotypes: q^2 X 100 =   0.13 X 0.13 X 100 = 1.69

As always check to see that the totals equal 100 (individuals in this case).

$$= 75.69 + 22.62 + 1.69 = \underline{100}$$

Test these data: $\chi^2 =$ $\displaystyle\sum \frac{(\text{observed numbers} - \text{expected numbers})^2}{\text{expected numbers}}$

χ^2 = $(75 - 75.69)^2 / 75.69$ + $(24 - 22.62)^2 / 22.62 +$ $(1 - 1.69)^2 / 1.69$

   = 0.54

It is now necessary to interpret the χ^2 value of 0.54 by examining a χ^2 table (given in your text). To do so, one needs to determine the number of degrees of freedom, which is based on the number of "free variables" typical of most statistical tests. However, the number of "free variables" in many significance tests of this type is reduced by an additional degree of freedom because while making the calculations, we estimated a parameter (p or q) to determine the expected values. Therefore, one degree of freedom is lost for estimating a parameter and one degree of freedom is lost for dealing with a fixed number of individuals (100 in this case). Even though there are three classes (*AA*, *AS*, and *SS*, n - 3), there will be n – 2 degrees of freedom when entering the χ^2 table. Checking the table with one degree of freedom gives a value of 3.84 at the 0.05 probability level. Since the χ^2 value calculated in this problem is smaller (0.54 < 3.84), the null hypothesis, that the observed values fluctuate from the HW expected values by chance and chance alone, should not be rejected. Therefore, the frequencies of *AA, AS,* and *SS* sampled a population of 100 individuals that is consistent with a population that is in a HW equilibrium.

Sentence 5 and answer (b): The population appears to be in a HW equilibrium, yet the question states that the sample of 100 individuals was taken from a relatively small, isolated population. Generally, in small, isolated populations either genetic drift or nonrandom mating occurs. The HW assumptions call for large, randomly mating populations. Perhaps the population sampled was only recently isolated, there is random mating with little drift, or the HW expectations occurred purely by chance.

Kritzik and colleagues (1998) discovered three alleles of the *alpha2* gene that influence blood platelet function and may be significant in thrombosis and/or bleeding in humans. Nucleotide substitutions account for variants *1*, *2*, and *3*. Assume the following variant frequencies in a given population from North America:

$$variant\ 1\ =\ 0.5$$
$$variant\ 2\ =\ 0.3$$
$$variant\ 3\ =\ 0.2$$

Given these values, of 1000 individuals sampled, what would be the predicted population distribution of genotypes under Hardy-Weinberg equilibrium assumptions?

Concepts/Processes in Question 4: This question requires an understanding and application of the **HW formula** for **multiple alleles**.

Analysis of Question 4:

A population genetics application to multiple alleles will be involved

Level 2. Kritzik and colleagues (1998) discovered three alleles of the *alpha2* gene that influence blood platelet function and may be significant in thrombosis and/or bleeding in humans.[1] Nucleotide substitutions account for variants *1*, *2*, and *3*.[2] Assume the following variant frequencies in a given population from North America:[3]

$$variant\ 1\ =\ 0.5$$
$$variant\ 2\ =\ 0.3$$
$$variant\ 3\ =\ 0.2$$

These genotypes should be various combinations of the three alleles, taken two at a time

Given these values, of 1000 individuals sampled, what would be the predicted population distribution of genotypes under Hardy-Weinberg equilibrium assumptions?[4]

Sentence 1: This sentence provides background and an indication of the significance of the work of Kritzik and colleagues. It has no direct influence on the solution to the question.

Sentence 2: The number of variants is provided along with the symbols. There are three variants in this multiple allelic series.

Sentence 3: The frequencies of the individual variants are provided. These values will be applied to the general formula for the distribution of HW equilibrium genotypes for multiple alleles given below.

Sentence 4 and answer: The general expressions for dealing with three alleles in a HW context are as follows:

allelic frequencies: $p + q + r = 1.0$

genotypic or zygotic frequencies:

$$p^2 + 2pq + q^2 + 2pr + 2qr + r^2 = 1.0$$

Substituting the values for p, q, and r stated in the problem gives the following genotypic distributions:

frequency of *1.1*	=	p^2	=	0.5 X 0.5	=	0.25
frequency of *1.2*	=	$2pq$	=	2(0.5 X 0.3)	=	0.30
frequency of *2.2*	=	q^2	=	0.3 X 0.3	=	0.09
frequency of *1.3*	=	$2pr$	=	2(0.5 X 0.2)	=	0.20
frequency of *2.3*	=	$2qr$	=	2(0.3 X 0.2)	=	0.12
frequency of *3.3*	=	r^2	=	0.2 X 0.2	=	0.04

Again, to be certain that all calculations are correct and all classes are accounted for, be certain that the total of the individual frequencies equals 1.0. Taking each frequency and multiplying by 1000 will give the expected distribution of individuals with each genotype.

number of *1.1* = 0.25 X 1000 = 250
number of *1.2* = 0.30 X 1000 = 300
number of *2.2* = 0.09 X 1000 = 90
number of *1.3* = 0.20 X 1000 = 200
number of *2.3* = 0.12 X 1000 = 120
number of *3.3* = 0.04 X 1000 = 40

A classic example of natural selection is the change of moth (*Biston betularia* and *Biston carbonaria*) coloration associated with industrialization in England. To quantify and predict changes in allelic frequency as a result of selection, a number of mathematical models have been developed. Assume that natural selection occurs against a recessive allele such that 50% of the homozygous recessive genotypes do not survive to reproduce.

(a) If the allelic frequencies in one generation of such a moth population are $p = 0.7$ and $q = 0.3$, what would be the allelic frequencies in the next generation?

(b) Would you expect the impact of such selection to be classified as *stabilizing*, *directional*, or *disruptive*?

Concepts/Processes in Question 5: This problem illustrates classic **selection against the homozygous recessive** group that causes a **directional change in genotypic frequencies**.

Predation on the light and dark forms of *Biston* led to changes in gene frequencies

A formula will allow an estimation of changes in allelic frequencies through time

Level 3: A classic example of natural selection is the change of moth (*Biston betularia* and *Biston carbonaria*) coloration associated with industrialization in England.[1] To quantify and predict changes in gene frequency as a result of selection, a number of mathematical models have been developed.[2] Assume that natural selection occurs against a recessive allele such that 50% of the homozygous recessive genotypes do not survive to reproduce.[3] **(a)** If the allelic frequencies in one generation of such a moth population are $p = 0.7$ and $q = 0.3$, what would be the allelic frequencies in the next generation?[4] **(b)** Would you expect the impact of such selection to be classified as *stabilizing*, *directional*, or *disruptive*?[5]

One would probably consider a significant drop in the frequency of the recessive gene over time

---

Sentence 1: As pollution darkened lichen-covered city surfaces in industrial areas in England, the lighter moths were more obvious to predators, and selection favored a darker form.

Sentence 2: The general mathematical model for selection against homozygous recessive individuals is as follows:

Genotype	*Fitness*
AA	1.0
Aa	1.0
aa	1.0 – selection coefficient

If *q* is the initial frequency of the recessive allele and *s* is the selection coefficient, then

$$q' = \frac{q - sq^2}{1 - sq^2}$$

is the frequency of the recessive allele in the next generation.

Sentence 3: Since only half of individuals that express the recessive allele survive to produce offspring, the selection coefficient is 0.5.

Sentence 4 and answer (a): Applying the selection coefficient of 0.5 to the equation with the other values substituted, gives the following answer.

$$q' = \frac{q - sq^2}{1 - sq^2}$$

$$q' = \frac{0.3 - 0.5(0.09)}{1 - 0.5(0.09)}$$

$$q' = 0.267$$

Sentence 5 and answer (b): There are generally three models that summarize the influence of selection on allelic frequencies: *stabilizing*, *directional*, and *disruptive*, as illustrated below (the dotted line represents the mean of an original population trait, and the solid line represents the mean population trait after selection). From the information given in this question, the allelic frequencies shift in one direction, away from *q* and toward *p*. Therefore, the directional model is favored.

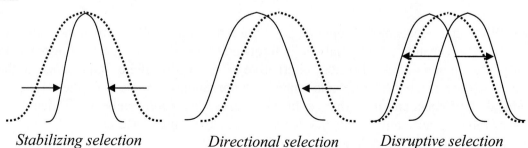

Stabilizing selection   *Directional selection*   *Disruptive selection*

Migration can be a strong force in evolution, especially if there are large differences in allelic frequencies and if the migrants are appreciable in number. Consider populations on two islands *A* and *B* in which members from island *B* often migrate to island *A*. Assume that the frequency of the *Clc* allele (of two alleles) on island *A* is 0.4 and on island *B* it is 0.6: p_A = 0.4, p_B = 0.6. Assume also that 20% of the breeding population for the next generation migrates from island *B* to island *A* and migrants randomly mate with members of island *A*. In the next generation, what will be the frequency of the *Clc* allele on island *A*?

Concepts/Processes in Question 6: This question addresses **changes in allelic frequency** due to **migration** and illustrates that the degree of change is directly related to the **number of migrants** and the **genetic differences** between populations.

Analysis of Question 6:

Migration is the movement of individuals from one population to another

Level 3. Migration can be a strong force in evolution, especially if there are large differences in allelic frequencies and if the migrants are appreciable in number.[1] Consider populations on two islands *A* and *B* in which members from island *B* often migrate to island *A*.[2] Assume that the frequency of the *Clc* allele (of two alleles) on island *A* is 0.4 and on island *B* it is 0.6: p_A = 0.4, p_B = 0.6.[3] Assume also that 20% of the breeding population for the next generation migrates from island *B* to island *A* and migrants randomly mate with members of island *A*.[4] In the next generation, what will be the frequency of the *Clc* allele on island *A*?[5]

Let the frequency of the *Clc* allele = *p*

Sentence 1: When individuals move from one population to another, allelic frequencies in the recipient population change if the initial allelic frequencies are different and the migrants are sufficiently large in number. A "flip side" alternative exists. If the allelic frequencies are the same in two populations, but the migrants represent a nonrandom sample from the originating population, allelic frequencies may change. In some cases, migration can be a significant evolutionary force because individuals that leave a given geographic area are usually not a random sample of the home population.

Sentence 2: Information in Sentence 2 is illustrated in the figure below:

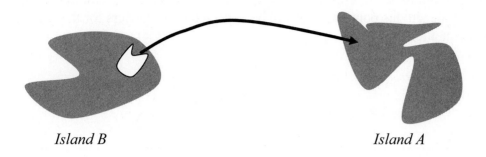

Island B   *Island A*

Sentences 3 and 4: The following graphic illustrates the allelic frequencies in both island populations.

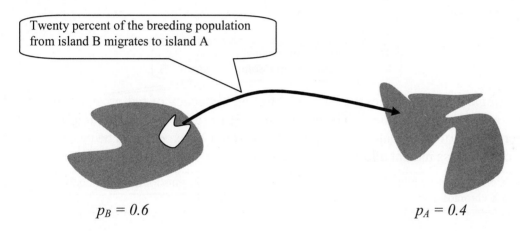

$p_B = 0.6$ $p_A = 0.4$

Sentences 5 and answer: The migration rate is symbolized by *m* (20%), and the new allelic frequency for the receiving population (on island *A*) in response to migration is given by the following formula:

$$P_{Anew} = (1 - m)p_A + mp_B$$

Substituting in values according to this example gives the following:

$$P_{Anew} = [(1 - 0.2) \times 0.4] + (0.2 \times 0.6)$$

$$P_{Anew} = 0.44$$

A large sample of human males was screened for the frequency of red-green color blindness, and 80 out of 1000 were found to be color-blind. If Hardy-Weinberg assumptions are satisfied, what percentage of the females in this population would be expected to be carriers for the red-green color blindness mutant allele?

Concepts/Processes in Question 7: This question addresses the estimation of **allelic frequencies for X-linked genes**.

Analysis of Question 7:

The red-green color blindness gene is located on the X chromosome in humans

Level 2. A large sample of human males was screened for the frequency of red-green color blindness, and 80 out of 1000 were found to be color-blind.[1] If Hardy-Weinberg assumptions are satisfied, what percentage of the females in this population would be expected to be carriers for the red-green color blindness mutant allele?[2]

Males have one X chromosome while females have two X chromosomes

Carriers are heterozygous for the trait in question

Sentence 1: The fact that the red-green color blindness is X-linked is not provided in this question. This could be an oversight by the author of the question or it is assumed that students would know that red-green color blindness is caused by an X-linked gene. Since 80 out of 1000 males are red-green color-blind, the frequency of the mutant allele is 0.08 or $q = 0.08$ and $p = 0.92$

Sentence 2 and answer: Since females have two X chromosomes, and the question asks for the percentage of heterozygous carriers, the following applies:

$$\text{frequency of heterozygotes} \ = \ 2pq \ = \ 2\,(0.92 \ \times \ 0.08) \ = \ 0.1472$$

Therefore 14.72 percent of the females in this population would be expected to be carriers of the red-green color blindness mutant allele.

Index

Index

Index

Index